Psychiatric Ethics in Late-Life Patients

W0050745

Meera Balasubramaniam
Aarti Gupta • Rajesh R. Tampi
Editors

Psychiatric Ethics in Late-Life Patients

Medicolegal and Forensic
Aspects at the Interface
of Mental Health

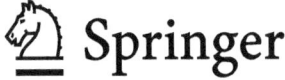 Springer

Editors
Meera Balasubramaniam
New York University School
of Medicine
New York, NY, USA

Aarti Gupta
Yale University School of
Medicine
New Haven, CT, USA

Rajesh R. Tampi
Yale School of Medicine
New Haven, CT, USA

Cleveland Clinic Lerner
College of Medicine of Case
Western Reserve University
Cleveland, OH, USA

ISBN 978-3-030-15171-3   ISBN 978-3-030-15172-0   (eBook)
https://doi.org/10.1007/978-3-030-15172-0

This Springer imprint is published by the registered company Springer Nature Switzerland AG
The registered company address is: Gewerbestrasse 11, 6330 Cham, Switzerland

Preface

The population of older adults in the United States is growing at a significant rate. It is estimated that by 2035, there will be 78.0 million people ≥65 years in age when compared to 76.7 million people ≤18 years in age. By 2060, the population of Americans ≥65 years in age is projected to increase from the current 46 million (15% of the population) to over 98 million (24% of the population).

It is estimated that one in five older adults in the United States has a diagnosable psychiatric and/or substance use disorder. Given the substantial increase in the number of older adults with mental health and substance use disorders in the recent decades, the healthcare system is becoming overburdened providing care for these individuals. In addition, the critical shortage of trained clinicians who are able to appropriately care for older adults with psychiatric and substance use disorders has resulted in provision of substandard care for this vulnerable population.

A significant number of older adults also face a multitude of medical, psychological, and social issues that impair their activities of daily living and worsen their quality of life. In addition, a considerable number of older adults also lose their independence and autonomy due to the presence of chronic medical and/or psychiatric disorders. Many of these individuals are vulnerable to exploitation and abuse given their cognitive, psychiatric, and physical impairments.

Psychiatric Ethics in Late-Life Patients: Medicolegal and Forensic Aspects at the Interface of Mental Health is a book that is written to provide the most up-to-date information of these topics. This book is meant for use by anyone who is involved with the care of older adults, be it a family member, a caregiver, a student, a trainee, a novice clinician, or a seasoned professional. The goal behind this project was to produce a concise and appropriately priced book which encompasses the latest information on ethical, medicolegal, and forensic issues among individuals in late life. It is written by experienced professionals who specialize in the care of older adults. We hope that the readers of this book will get as much satisfaction from reading this volume as we had in writing it for them.

New York, NY, USA   Meera Balasubramaniam, MD, MPH
New Haven, CT, USA   Aarti Gupta, MD
New Haven, CT, USA   Rajesh R. Tampi, MD, MS,
Cleveland, OH, USA   DFAPA, DFAAGP

Contents

Contributors

Ali Abbas Asghar-Ali, MD VA South Central Mental Illness Research, Education and Clinical Center, Houston, TX, USA

VA HSR&D Center for Innovations in Quality, Effectiveness and Safety, Michael E. DeBakey VA Medical Center, Houston, TX, USA

Department of Psychiatry, Baylor College of Medicine, Houston, TX, USA

Meera Balasubramaniam, MD, MPH New York University School of Medicine, New York, NY, USA

Jennifer Bryan, PhD VA South Central Mental Illness Research, Education and Clinical Center, Houston, TX, USA

VA HSR&D Center for Innovations in Quality, Effectiveness and Safety, Michael E. DeBakey VA Medical Center, Houston, TX, USA

Department of Psychiatry, Baylor College of Medicine, Houston, TX, USA

Mary E. Camp, MD University of Texas Southwestern Medical Center, Dallas, TX, USA

Alexander Cole, MD University of Texas Southwestern Medical Center, Dallas, TX, USA

Jeremy Colley, MD Department of Psychiatry, New York University School of Medicine, New York, NY, USA

Dhweeja Dasarathy Harvard University, Cambridge, MA, USA

Romika Dhar, MD Department of Medicine, West Virginia University School of Medicine, Morgantown, WV, USA

Nery A. Diaz, DO Columbia University Irving Medical Center, New York, NY, USA

New York State Psychiatric Institute, New York, NY, USA

Laura B. Dunn, MD Department of Psychiatry and Behavioral Sciences, Stanford University, Stanford, CA, USA

Reiko Emtman, MD Boise VA Medical Center, Boise, ID, USA

Oliver M. Glass, MD Emory University, Department of Psychiatry and Behavioral Sciences, Atlanta, GA, USA

Aarti Gupta, MD Yale University School of Medicine, New Haven, CT, USA

Adriana P. Hermida, MD Emory University, Department of Psychiatry and Behavioral Sciences, Atlanta, GA, USA

Rakin Hoq, MD Department of Psychiatry, Summa Health System, Akron, OH, USA

Adriana Kaye, BA, MSW Candidate Fordham University Graduate School of Social Services, New York, NY, USA

Sarah A. Kleinfeld, MD Washington, DC VA Medical Center, Washington, DC, USA

Jananie Kumaran, MD Department of Psychiatry, Saskatchewan Health Authority, Saskatoon, SK, Canada

Department of Psychiatry, Saskatchewan College of Medicine, Saskatoon, SK, Canada

Feyza Marouf, MD Massachusetts General Hospital, Boston, MA, USA

Harvard Medical School, Boston, MA, USA

Tina Maschi, PhD, LCSW, ACSW Fordham University Graduate School of Social Services, New York, NY, USA

Reema D. Mehta, MD Jacobi Medical Center, Bronx, NY, USA

Albert Einstein College of Medicine, Bronx, NY, USA

Rohini Mehta, MD Medstar Georgetown University Hospital, Washington, DC, USA

Sabrina Pickens, PhD, MSN, GNP-BC, ANP-BC Cizik School of Nursing, The University of Texas Health Science Center, Houston, TX, USA

Monika Pietrzak, JD New York University School of Medicine, New York, NY, USA

Iuliana Predescu, MD UPMC Altoona, Altoona, PA, USA

Mary Ellen Trail Ross, DrPH, MSN, RN, GCNS-BC Cizik School of Nursing, The University of Texas Health Science Center, Houston, TX, USA

Jason Strauss, MD Cambridge Health Alliance, Harvard Medical School, Everett, MA, USA

Bipin Subedi, MD Department of Psychiatry, New York University School of Medicine, New York, NY, USA

Katharine L. Thomas Rice University, Houston, TX, USA

Larry Tune, MD Emory University, Department of Psychiatry and Behavioral Sciences, Atlanta, GA, USA

Edward J. Wicht, MD, JD, LLM Private Practice, Washington, DC, USA

Part I
Ethical Aspects
of Geriatric Psychiatry

Chapter 1
Aging: Balancing Autonomy and Beneficence

Reiko Emtman and Jason Strauss

Introduction

The "silver tsunami" is approaching. In 2014, there were 46 million people in the United States over the age of 65; 6 million of those were age 85 and older. By 2060, the number of individuals over age 65 will more than double to 98 million, and the number of individuals over age 85 will more than triple to 20 million [15]. In addition, the number of older adults with psychiatric and substance use disorder continues to increase at an appreciable rate. According to the Institute of Medicine (IOM), by 2030, expected growth in the older population will increase the number of older people with mental health and substance use conditions by 80% [12]. Moving forward, medical providers will be asked to confront an increasing number of challenges in navigating our professional desire to be as helpful as possible to

———
R. Emtman
Boise VA Medical Center, Boise, ID, USA
e-mail: Reiko.emtman@va.gov

J. Strauss (✉)
Cambridge Health Alliance, Harvard Medical School,
Everett, MA, USA
e-mail: jbstrauss@challiance.org

© Springer Nature Switzerland AG 2019
M. Balasubramaniam et al. (eds.), *Psychiatric Ethics in Late-Life Patients*, https://doi.org/10.1007/978-3-030-15172-0_1

3

our older patients when our recommendations do not align with their wishes.

As healthcare systems and providers strive to address the needs of an aging population, it is important to consider the potential impacts of aging on individual autonomy. Autonomy is freedom from external control or influence and is often considered synonymous with independence [2]. In the care of older adults, practitioners frequently encounter individuals who value and prioritize maintaining autonomy. Beneficence is defined as an action done to benefit others and has connotations of mercy, kindness, and promoting the good of others [2]. Benevolence is sometimes used to justify paternalism, or the concept that renders acceptable attempts to benefit another person, even when the other person does not prefer to receive benefit. Historically, physicians delivered medical care in a paternalistic way, where the expected dynamic in the healthcare relationship assigned authority and expertise to the physician, who provided education, recommendations, and advice to the patient [3].

Today's healthcare system is moving away from a paternalistic model and toward self-management [3]. In this model, the focus of the clinical encounter is to teach problem-solving skills and promote patient self-efficacy as a way of managing chronic medical illnesses [3]. In working together to manage chronic disease collaboratively, the patient and the provider work toward patient-identified goals, which can have ego-syntonic effects even in the context of chronic illness.

The growing pains of this paradigm shift are reflected in the struggles of medical specialists adopting new terminology to refer to patients [19]. Psychiatry has struggled with whether to refer to individuals seeking psychiatric care as patients, as most of their medical colleagues do, or as clients, as is becoming more common among their mental health colleagues in psychology and social work [26]. A similar struggle has emerged for how to respectfully describe individuals who are farther along on the aging continuum: "older adults," "elderly," "geriatric," "seniors," "aged," and the "young-old" *versus* "old-old" [11].

Ethical Frameworks in Medicine and Research: Integration of Autonomy and Beneficence

Several key frameworks are helpful in providing context for the discussion of autonomy and beneficence in older adults. In caring for older adults who commonly have multiple disease states in addition to physiologic changes with aging, the principles of autonomy and beneficence can come into conflict with one another [2, 5, 14, 20]. Clinical examples of conflicts between autonomy and beneficence will be discussed later in this chapter. Table 1.1 provides a comparison of four commonly used ethics frameworks for approaching issues that arise in the course of clinical practice.

A detailed review of each of these ethical frameworks is outside the scope of this chapter. Table 1.1 compares four such frameworks. A brief introduction to each of the aforementioned models will be presented here. The moral principles outlined by Beauchamp and Childress [2] have been longstanding pillars in the realm of medical ethics [14]. Jonsen et al. designed a framework for medical profession-

TABLE 1.1 Ethical frameworks considering autonomy and beneficence

Moral Principles By Beauchamp & Childress	The Four Topics By Jonsen, Seigler & Winslade	Fundamental Principles From the Charter on Medical Professionalism	Ethical Principles in Human Subjects Research From The Belmont Report
Respect for Autonomy	Medical Indications	Patient Welfare	Respect for Persons
Nonmaleficence	Patient Preferences	Patient Autonomy	Beneficence
Beneficence	Quality of Life	Social Justice	Justice
Justice	Contextual Features		
Professional-Patient Relationships			
Legend:			
☐ Principle emphasizing or stemming from autonomy			
■ Principle emphasizing or stemming from beneficence			

als and professionals within the healthcare system to provide a practical approach to solving ethical issues that arise in the practice of medicine. The Charter on Medical professionalism, published in 2002, was designed to address ethical conflicts that arise in the context of healthcare systems in the new millennium and renew physicians' commitments to the welfare of patients [5]. In 1974, the National Research Act became law, which created the National Commission for the Protection of Human Subjects of Biomedical and Behavioral Research. The product of this commission, entitled The Belmont Report, outlined ethical principles pertaining to biomedical and behavioral research involving human subjects [20].

Next, we will examine the principle of autonomy as presented in each of these four frameworks. Figure 1.1 provides a concise summary of autonomy as presented in each framework.

In the practice of geriatrics, how far should clinicians go to respect autonomy of a patient? Under what circumstances is a paternalistic approach acceptable? Older adults will have varying degrees of decisional capacity, but it is important to recognize the distinction between autonomy and decisional

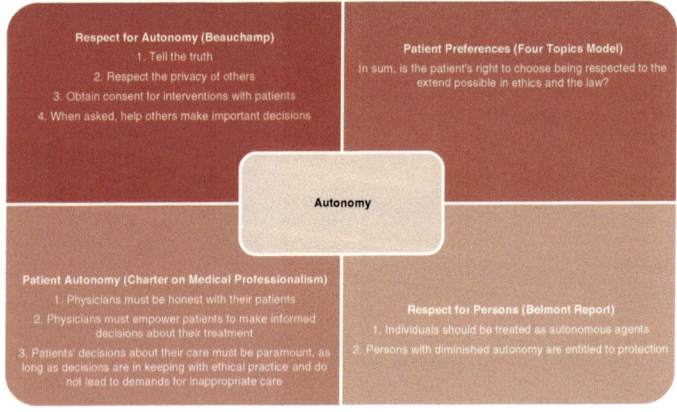

FIGURE 1.1 Ethical frameworks of autonomy

capacity. Even individuals who lack the capability to make autonomous decisions can still make autonomous choices [13]. For example, an older adult who does not have the decisional capacity to refuse placement in a short-term rehabilitation facility can still make autonomous choices about meal preferences, choices about their daily routine, their level of participation in activities and whether to initiate social contact with others. Clinicians show respect for patient autonomy through their actions and clinical decision-making and should frame any treatment recommendations in terms of how each recommendation fits into helping the patient achieve their goals. Respecting autonomy requires clinicians to refrain from obstructing a patient's right to make their own determinations or judgments [2]. Patient preferences incorporate the spirit of autonomy, without having the connotation that an individual must have decisional capacity for complete self-determination and instead shifts the focus to allowing choice wherever reasonable. A paternalistic approach that overrides patient autonomy is indicated when a person's preferences and actions infringe on the rights and/or welfare of another individual. In geriatrics, autonomy may need to be overridden to protect the safety of family or professional caregivers, other residents in a facility and the health of the public.

The principle of beneficence is a universal goal of the healthcare system [2, 14]. Here, we will examine factors that can impede principles of beneficence in clinical practice and discuss the role of mental health providers in some common situations. These principles are also compared in Fig. 1.2. One example of this is when patients or their family members request medically inappropriate treatment. An example of this is the use of feeding tubes to treat dysphagia resulting from advanced dementia. Given the social, cultural, and sometimes religious significance of eating and sharing food, families can experience distress when their loved one is no longer able to eat, and request feeding tube placement. However, studies have shown that feeding tubes do not provide survival benefit when used in patients with advanced

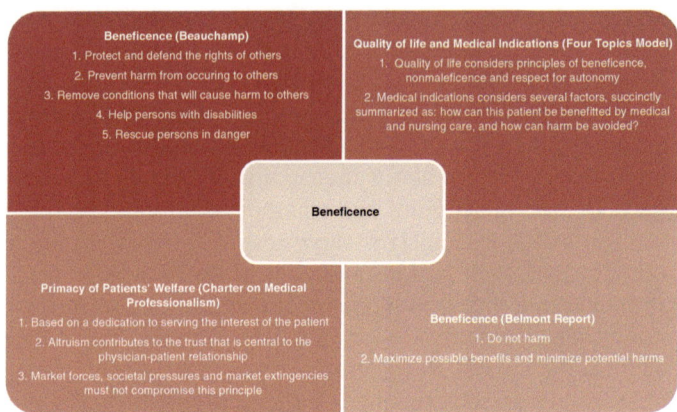

FIGURE 1.2 Ethical frameworks of beneficence

dementia and that use of feeding tubes is associated with higher rates of agitation, chemical, and physical restraint [1]. Another common clinical scenario when it can be difficult for providers to practice benevolence is in patients with severe personality disorders. Research shows that adults with personality disorders have a reduced life expectancy, which may be due to difficulties with interfacing effectively with healthcare systems [10, 22].

Physiologic Changes of Aging that Can Impact Autonomy

In this section, we will take an organ-systems approach to examine physiologic changes of aging that can contribute to decreased independence and recommend ways that psychiatric practice can promote autonomy. In order to provide optimal care for older adults, clinicians must integrate an understanding of the physiologic changes that occur with aging into their treatment plans and make appropriate referrals to interdisciplinary healthcare providers and subspecialists when indicated [16].

Physiologic changes that occur within the central nervous system with aging include a decrease in the number of neurotransmitters and their corresponding receptors, decreased dendritic branches at the neuronal level and formation of extracellular tangles and intracellular plaques [21]. Clinicians must remain vigilant about screening for psychiatric conditions that impact individuals of all ages: mood disorders, anxiety disorders, psychotic disorders, and substance use disorders and also pay close attention to domains of attention and cognition during an encounter with an older adult [6]. It is important to consider depression and pseudodementia on the differential diagnosis for individuals who appear to have cognitive deficits [8]. Individuals who have severe cognitive impairment tend to lose a degree of autonomy when another individual assumes a power of attorney or guardianship, but confidentiality and choice should be respected to the extent that is possible. Psychiatric providers should maintain a high degree of suspicion for medial etiologies of psychiatric illness and should have an understanding of psychiatric side effects of medical treatments as they may cause cognitive and functional impairments which can impede an individual's autonomy [9].

Sensory impairment can have a significant impact on autonomy in older adults [7]. Clinicians should inquire about vision and hearing and refer to optometry, ophthalmology, and audiology as appropriate. An opportunity for clinicians to act in a beneficent manner in any setting is to maintain an environmental awareness and promptly address or report hazards such as wet floors, uneven surfaces to appropriate personnel to minimize the potential for accidents such as falls for individuals who, because of sensory limitations, are vulnerable to injury from environmental hazards.

Mobility issues can have a substantial impact on wellbeing and independence [18]. Physiologic changes of aging impact the musculoskeletal system and include sarcopenia, degenerative joint disease, osteopenia, and pathologic osteoporosis. These changes can increase the risk for falls and the likelihood of serious injury resulting from a fall. The benevolent psychiatric provider should be mindful about weighing benefits of psychiatric medications against potential for fall risk and ensuring appropriate referrals are placed for evaluation of home safety, strength, balance, and mobility issues as indicated. Neurophysiologic changes that occur with aging and often contribute to aforementioned issues with mobility include peripheral neuropathy, potential weakness from prior cerebrovascular accident(s), diminished reflexes, and slowed reaction time.

The physiology of aging in the cardiovascular system should also be taken into account when prescribing psychiatric medications [17]. Certain psychiatric medications can increase the risk of orthostatic hypotension and cardiac arrhythmias, which should be taken into consideration prior to initiating medication changes in older adults. The importance of collaborating with primary care providers and appropriate specialists cannot be overemphasized [25].

In the practice of geriatrics, clinicians must be able to apply the physiologic mechanisms of aging and combine the knowledge with clinical assessment of instrumental activities of daily living (ADLs), social supports, and quality of life to reach sound clinical decisions and offer medically appropriate interventions while withholding interventions that are unlikely to lead to achievement of a patient's healthcare goals. Decisions regarding medical indications can be guided by use of frailty indexes which in turn, may improve beneficence of medical care offered and delivered, and offer a tool for prognostication [16].

Autonomy in the Clinical Encounter

Translating theoretical principles of autonomy into concrete action during a clinical encounter requires habitual incorporation of patient-centered communication styles. Table 1.2 examines ways in which the clinical encounter itself can foster or weaken autonomy.

TABLE 1.2 Examining autonomy in the clinical encounter

	Reinforces autonomy	**Undermines autonomy**
Setting the frame	Identify relationship/ role of all individuals present. Seek the client's consent to have family member/ caregiver join the visit	Begin the visit without acknowledging all parties present and their role/relationship
	Begin by asking the client what their concerns are, set agenda together	Allowing only agenda items brought up by the provider or family member/caregiver
	Ask patient for permission to obtain information from caregiver/family member	Interact with family member as though client is not present
	Seek assent to speak with client and family member separately in some circumstances, giving both parties individual time with provider	Ask client to leave the room while provider talks to family member
Linguistics	Refer to client in second person, i.e. "your reaction to x"	Refer to client in third person, i.e., "his behaviors"
Body language	Provider spends most of the encounter facing client	Provider spends most of the encounter facing family member/ caregiver
	Provider maintains eye contact primarily with patient when discussing treatment plan and recommendations	Provider maintains eye contact primarily with the family member/caregiver when discussing treatment plan and recommendations

(continued)

TABLE I.2 (continued)

	Reinforces autonomy	**Undermines autonomy**
Concluding the visit	Begin by asking client what questions they have	Only ask family member/caregiver if they have questions
	Discuss recommendations and treatment plan using straight forward, second person language	Outline recommendations and treatment plan quickly, using jargon and third person language
	Thank the client for allowing provider and family member/caregiver to work with them	Thank family member/caregiver for bringing client to the appointment

There are several tools available to guide practitioners to facilitate a discussion about an individual's wishes in hopes of preserving autonomy (Conversation Started Kit, [24]). In the United States, individuals can indicate their preferences regarding specific life-sustaining medical interventions such as cardiopulmonary resuscitation, artificial nutrition and hydration, and antibiotic use, among others. This document is known as an advance directive [4]. Individuals can also appoint a surrogate decision-maker who they have identified to make decisions about their medical care in the event that they are incapable of doing so themselves.

In addition to the legal methods that an individual can make their healthcare preferences known, clinicians should be aware of available clinical tools that can serve as a guide for providers to explore an individual patient's values, and for patients to obtain information about their healthcare condition and its prognosis from their providers. Table 1.3 provides an example of tools that can be used to facilitate discussion with patients in the clinical setting (Conversation Starter Kit, [24]). The use of such tools can serve as a guide for surrogate decision-makers and providers, which can be a step toward preservation of autonomy.

TABLE 1.3 Clinical tools used to facilitate discussion of autonomy in making healthcare decisions

Tool	Description
The Conversation Starter Kit	12-page informational guide providing education about the importance of communicating end of life wishes and a concrete action plan
Created by the Conversation Project and the Institute for Healthcare Improvement
Available in 11 languages
Values Questionnaire	10 open-ended questions to help individuals think about values as they relate to healthcare decisions
Created by the Vermont Ethics Network

Beneficence in Clinical Practice

In addition to providing compassionate, evidence-based psychiatric care, psychiatrists providing care for older adults should be mindful of the team-based nature of healthcare for older adults [23]. Collaboration and communication with interdisciplinary members of the medical team are key, and psychiatrists can offer guidance on how to handle manifestations of personality disorders, characterological traits, and disinhibited behaviors, to name a few.

A familiarity with community and systemic supports designed to support older adults as they face common age-associated challenges available in the community is beneficial. Older adults can maintain autonomy and see benefits in their quality of life by utilizing programs and services such as adult day health, home caregivers, and senior transit options. Referral to caregiver support programs is another area that psychiatrists should be comfortable speaking to.

Beneficent behavior exists outside of the clinical encounter: alerting facility staff of environmental hazards that could lead to injury or falls and stopping to give directions to individuals who appear lost are common manifestations of beneficence on a healthcare campus.

Healthcare systems must adapt to needs of the older population and must take environmental concerns into account to care for an aging population: clinics for older adults must have relatively close proximity to a parking lot to be accessible to individuals with mobility limitations. Ways to deliver interdisciplinary healthcare to older adults in their home make these services accessible to a larger population.

Situations Where Autonomy and Beneficence May Conflict in Older Adults

Case #1

Mr. D is an 83-year-old male with depression, minor neuro-cognitive disorder, and hoarding disorder. He has been living at his skilled nursing facility for the past 2 years, after he was evicted from his senior housing in the community for repeated safety violations related to his hoarding disorder. Mr. D is generally well-liked by staff at the nursing facility, which he shares with two peers who are significantly more cognitively impaired than he is. Mr. D is noted to be pleasant and adherent with medications and daily care. He enjoys reading and spends time in the periphery of the milieu of his unit. However, he becomes passively suicidal, irritable, and occasionally combative with staff when his room is scheduled for its monthly cleaning. On one occasion, he was so distressed that he required inpatient psychiatric hospitalization. These behaviors have led to his being on escalating doses of antipsychotic medications.

Case #2

Ms. T is a 77-year-old female with chronic paranoid schizophrenia. She resides on a locked "behavioral" unit of a skilled nursing facility. Prior to transitioning to this facility, she had lived by herself. She never married, had few friends, and she had not kept in touch with family for many years. She worked from home and enjoyed participating in solitary activities. Ms. T has functionally declined and has become incontinent of bowel and urine. She has become increasingly reluctant to allow staff to provide any kind of care to her. She declines to bathe and will not partake in any attempts at grooming. Ultimately, she refuses to change her clothes even as they become increasingly soiled. Staff suspects that she has growing pressure ulcers at risk of being infected, but Ms. T refuses to allow her caregivers to check for them. She never becomes irritable or combative, but her resistance to care increases. Adjustments have been made to her antipsychotic regimen, but the behaviors have persisted. Peers on the unit (especially her two roommates) have noted the foul odor emanating from the room. In several cases, the smell has caused significant distress leading to worsening behavioral symptoms. Staff at the facility are increasingly reluctant to work with her and there is strong sentiment to psychiatrically hospitalize her.

Case #3

Mr. P is a 71-year-old male with post-traumatic stress disorder and major depressive disorder. He has chronic obstructive pulmonary disorder and must use oxygen through a nasal cannula. He lives alone in an apartment in a senior housing complex. He states that the only thing that brings him comfort is smoking, although there are strict building rules against doing this in his apartment. He was threatened with eviction following his second hospital admission in the past 3 months for pneumonia. He adamantly refuses to use a nicotine patch or gum and will not consider other interventions to curb his smoking. While he states that he understands the risks that his smoking presents to himself and others, he declines to change his behaviors. "I'd rather be homeless than live here and not be able to smoke."

Case #4

Ms. S is a 62-year-old woman who is in a short-term rehabilitation facility. She was recently hospitalized for a right arm cellulitis which was felt to be related to her longstanding intravenous heroin use. She currently has a peripherally inserted central catheter (PICC) so that she can receive antibiotics for the next 4 weeks without having to consistently change peripheral lines. Within 48 hours of admission, Ms. S demands to leave the facility against medical advice. She is adamant that her pain is not being adequately managed. "I'd be better off anywhere but here."

Discussion

These disparate cases highlight just a few of the myriad ways in which individual autonomy may be in conflict with what others believe is best for these individuals and their surrounding environments. In each of these situations, the goal is for all parties to work together to find some mutually satisfactory common ground.

In Case #1, Mr. D's hoarding disorder has already led to significant adverse consequences, yet the behavior persists. How can staff at Mr. D's nursing facility work with him to relieve his anxiety and distress around his room cleanings which must occur for the safety and benefit of his roommates? He asks for a private room, which is not available. However, providing Mr. D with sufficient advanced notice (and friendly reminders) of when his room must be cleaned and allowing him to choose a fixed number of items designated for keeping may contribute to his having more control over this harrowing but necessary process.

Ms. T's situation in Case #2 is similar to Mr. D's in that an individual's decisions are having a profoundly deleterious impact on the surrounding environment. How can staff at her nursing facility treat Ms. T with respect while working with her to help regain the dignity that comes with cleanliness? Staff will likely have to perform intricate detective work to learn as much as possible about Ms. T's interests and habits to find ways to help her feel more comfortable to receive care. Is there a particular staff member that Ms. T seems to trust more than others to provide care? Perhaps there is someone in the outside community who can be enlisted to improve the situation. There may be an activity that Ms. T will be motivated to be part of.

In Case #3, Mr. P realizes the danger that his smoking presents yet he feels compelled to continue engaging in this behavior. Once again, it is crucial to try to understand Mr. P's actions. Perhaps he has engaged in smoking cessation treatments in the past and has been unsuccessful. He may find the prospect of another failure so shameful that he is reluctant to try again. Another possibility is that his participation in such a potentially self-destructive behavior is a manifestation of a depressive episode which can be addressed with psychotherapy and/or psychopharmacologic treatments. It may also be worth brainstorming with Mr. P to see if his smoking may be replaced by a less potentially harmful activity.

Ms. S presents the staff at her facility with the harrowing prospect of her heading for the streets craving heroin with an exposed PICC line in Case #4. Fortunately, we can think quickly to intervene. While it is common and for staff and caregivers to harbor countertransference toward substance users, it is crucial to push through such preconceptions and find out how the facility can better serve Ms. S's needs. An increased number of skilled nursing facilities are caring for older adults with substance use issues, and she should be offered counseling and assurance that her pain is being adequately but safely managed. An increased number of facilities are licensed to prescribe buprenorphine for treatment of substance use disorders. Regardless of her history and current presentation, Ms. S should be treated as respectfully as her peers.

Conclusions

Our aging population will lead to a litany of new and expanding challenges for medical providers to consider. It is a struggle for healthcare professionals when their recommendations do not line up with the wishes of their patients. This chapter has provided theoretical frameworks with which to consider ways to integrate patient autonomy and treater beneficence while providing examples in clinical practice of when these two concepts are not easily reconciled. Examples of clinical tools with which to broach this topic during the patient encounter were provided. Indeed, it will be crucial for medical providers to develop a more sophisticated understanding of the relationship between provider beneficence and patient autonomy to develop algorithms for handling situations in which the two are not in alignment.

References

1. American Society. American Geriatrics Society feeding tubes in advanced dementia position statement. JAGS. 2014;62(8): 1590–3.
2. Beauchamp TL, Childress JF. Principles of biomedical ethics. 6th ed. New York: Oxford University Press; 2009.
3. Bodenheimer T, Lorig K, Holman H, Grumbach K. Patient self-management of chronic disease in primary care. JAMA. 2002;288(19):2469–75.
4. Bradley EH, Wetle T, Horwitz SM. The patient self-determination act and advance directive completion in nursing homes. Arch Fam Med. 1998;7(5):417–23.
5. Brennan T, Blank L, Kimball H, Smelser N, Copeland R, Lavizzo R, et al. Medical professionalism in the new millennium: a physicians' charter. Lancet. 2002;359(9305):520–2.
6. Brodaty H, Low LF, Gibson L, Burns K. What is the best dementia screening instrument for general practiioners to use? Am J Psychiatry. 2006;14(5):391–400. https://doi.org/10.1097/01. JGP.0000216181.20416.b2.
7. Chaudry SI, McAvay G, Ning Y, Allore HG, Newman AB, Gill TM. Geriatric impairments and disability: the cardiovascular health study. J Am Geriatr Soc. 2010;58(9):1686–92. https://doi. org/10.1111/j.1532-5415.2010.03022.x.
8. Connors MH, Quinto L, Brodaty H. Longitudinal outcomes of patients with pseudodementia: a systematic review. Psychol Med. 2018;15:1–11.

9. Fick DM, Semla TP, Beizer J, Brandt N, Dombrowski R, DuBeau CE, et al. American Geriatrics Society 2015 updated beers criteria for potentially inappropriate medication use in older adults. J Am Geriatr Soc. 2015;63(11):2227–45. https://doi.org/10.1111/jgs.13702.

10. Fok ML, Hayes RD, Chang CK, Stewart R, Callard FJ, Moran P. Life expectancy at birth and all=cause mortality among people with personality disorder. J Psychosom Res. 2012;73(2):104–7. https://doi.org/10.1016/j.jpsychores.2012.05.001.

11. Graham J. The new old age: 'Elderly' No More. The New York Times. 2012. https://newoldage.blogs.nytimes.com/2012/04/19/elderly-no-more/. Accessed 29 Apr 2018.

12. Institute of Medicine. The mental health and substance use workforce for older adults: in whose hands? Washington, DC: The National Academies Press; 2012. https://doi.org/10.17226/13400.

13. Jacobs ML, Snow AL, Allen RS, Hartman CW, et al. Supporting autonomy in long-term care: lessons from nursing assistants. Geriatr Nurs. 2018;pii: S0197–4572:30186–1. https://doi.org/10.1016/j.gerinurse.2018.07.004.

14. Jonsen AR, Siegler M, Winslade WJ. Clinical ethics: a practical approach to ethical decisions in clinical medicine. 5th ed. New York: McGraw Hill; 2002.

15. Mather M, Jacobsen LA, Pollard KM. Aging in the United States. Population Bulletin. 2015;70(2):2–3.

16. Morley J, Vellas B, van Kan GA, Anker SD, Bauer JM, Bernabei R, et al. Frailty consensus: a call to action. J Am Med Dir Assoc. 2013;14(6):392–7. https://doi.org/10.1016/j.jamda.2013.03.022.

17. North BJ, Sinclair DA. The intersection between aging and cardiovascular disease. Circ Res. 2012;110(8):1097–108. https://doi.org/10.1161/CIRCRESAHA.111.246876.

18. Pedersen MM, Holt NE, Grand L, Kulinski LA, Beauchamp MK, Kiely DK, et al. Mild cognitive impairment status an mobility performance: an analysis from the Boston RISE study. J Gerontol A Biol Sci Med Sci. 2014;69(12):1511–8. https://doi.org/10.1093/gerona/glu063.

19. Ratnapalan S. Shades of grey: patient versus client. CMAJ. 2009;180(4):472. https://doi.org/10.1503/cmaj.081694.

20. Ryan KJ, Brady JV, Cooke RE, Height DI, Jonsen AR, King P, et al. The Belmont Report. The National Commission for the Protection of Human Subjects. 1979.

21. Sarlak G, Jenwitheesuk A, Chetsawang B, Govitrapong P. Effects of melatonin on nervous system aging. J Pharmacol Sci. 2013;123(1):9–24. https://doi.org/10.1254/jphs.13R01SR.
22. Tyrer P, Reed GM, Crawford MJ. Classification, assessment, prevalence, and effect of personality disorder. Lancet. 2015;385(9969):717–26. https://doi.org/10.1016/S0140-6736(14)61995-4.
23. Unutzer J, Katon W, Callahan CM, Williams JW Jr, Hunkeler E, Harpole L, et al. Collaborative care management of late-life depression in the primary care setting: a randomized controlled trial. JAMA. 2002;288(22):2836–45. Starter Kits. In: The Conversation Project/Institute for Healthcare Improvement. 2017. https://theconversationproject.org/starter-kits/ Accessed 01 May 2018.
24. Values Questionnaire. Vermont Ethics Network. 2018. http://www.vtethicsnetwork.org/downloads/patient-values-questionnaire-2018.pdf. Accessed 01 May 2018.
25. Wild B, Heider D, Maatouk I, Slaets J, Konig HH, Niehoff D, et al. Significance and costs of complex biopsychosocial healthcare needs in elderly people: results of a population-based study. Psychosom Med. 2014;76(7):497–502. https://doi.org/10.1097/PSY.0000000000000080.
26. Zeller S. 'Patient' vs. 'Client': how semantics influences the practice of psychiatry. Psychiatry Advisor. 2015. Available at: https://www.psychiatryadvisor.com/practice-management/semantics-influuences-practice-psychiatry/article/423869/3/. Accessed 29 Apr 2018.

Chapter 2
The Capacity to Make Medical Decisions

Sarah A. Kleinfeld, Rohini Mehta, and Edward J. Wicht

Introduction

Healthcare providers assess patients' medical decision capacity during every interaction, either implicitly or explicitly. This chapter examines the core components of a capacity determination, the consequences of a determining a patient's lack of capacity, and issues commonly arising in clinical practice, specifically focusing on elderly individuals and those with dementia. Evidence-based tools assessing cognition and capacity are also examined.

S. A. Kleinfeld (✉)
Washington, DC VA Medical Center,
Washington, DC, USA
e-mail: sarah.kleinfeld2@va.gov

R. Mehta
Medstar Georgetown University Hospital, Washington, DC, USA
e-mail: rohini.s.mehta@gunet.georgetown.edu

E. J. Wicht
Private Practice, Washington, DC, USA
e-mail: edward.wicht@medstar.net

© Springer Nature Switzerland AG 2019   21
M. Balasubramaniam et al. (eds.), *Psychiatric Ethics in Late-Life Patients*, https://doi.org/10.1007/978-3-030-15172-0_2

Components of a Capacity Assessment

Decision-making capacity comprises four key components : (1) a basic understanding of the relevant medical background and circumstances (2); an appreciation of the risks, benefits, and consequences of possible choices (3); the ability to communicate a choice; and (4) communicating the rationale for arriving at that decision [1]. It is noteworthy that capacity and competency are technically very different things. Determining a patient's medical decision-making capacity is a clinical assessment performed by clinicians. This is in contrast to a competency determination, which is a legal conclusion reached by a judge. Notwithstanding this distinction, the terms are often used interchangeably [2].

A crucial element of informed consent is the patient's understanding of the relevant information relating to his or her treatment. Ways in which healthcare providers may assess understanding include retrieval of key facts or data and repetition of this information in the correct order. Patients may also be asked to make interpretations based on information presented. Part of ensuring that patients are able to understand relevant data and their consequences relies on providers presenting this information in ways that are simple and easy to understand. Some assessors of capacity may choose to be present while the treating physician is explaining the relevant medical information to the patient, to ensure all parties understood what was discussed.

Appreciating the situation then lends itself to an evaluation of an understanding of the consequences of accepting or rejecting a choice. Ways in which providers may assess for this include asking patients to repeat why this choice is being recommended by their treater and the most likely result of each choice.

The communication of a choice, though it may seem obvious, is a key element of a capacity determination. Not only does the selected choice need to be clear, but the patient must be consistent in this determination. In other words, recurrent vacillations between healthcare decisions would suggest a patient is not communicating a clear, consistent choice. This is not to say that a patient lacks capacity if he changes his mind, but "repeated reversals" may be indicative of impairment [1].

Finally, the rationale for arriving at a treatment decision is highly subjective and patient specific. This is where patient values and treatment goals will be most apparent. The goal of the provider performing the capacity assessment will be to determine if a patient is weighing the risks against the benefits and arriving at a decision that is in line with his or her value system. Appelbaum and Grisso refer to this process as "examining the patient's chain of reasoning" [1].

Making a Determination of Lack of Capacity

Determining that a patient lacks capacity, that is, "incapacitated," removes the patient as a decision-maker. If the patient has an advanced directive or healthcare power of attorney, decision-making duties revert to the patient's previously designated surrogate decision-maker. If no such document exists (and data suggest that despite clinician's efforts to persuade patients to prepare such documents very few patients actually have them), decision-making authority goes to a surrogate decision-maker according to a statutorily established hierarchy which ranks various family relations. Rankings vary some from state to state, but spouses are typically ranked first.

In some cases, incapacitated adult patients also lack family or a previously designated legal appointee. For these so-called unbefriended adults, the American Geriatric Society (AGS) encourages clinicians to utilize non-traditional surrogates, such as a non-married partner, close friends, members of a religious group, or even neighbors. AGS encourages clinicians to actively work to find a suitable non-traditional surrogate whenever possible. If a non-traditional surrogate cannot be identified, another avenue is to obtain a long-term surrogate who is familiar with the clinically relevant facts of a patient's care, usually in the form of a court-appointed legal guardian [3]. While a variety of approaches may be taken,

AGS recommends healthcare institutions to develop clear policies that are implemented consistently in accordance with state law.

A unique situation to consider arises when an unbe-friended adult lacks capacity in an emergency situation. AGS encourages healthcare entities to establish clear and consis-tent policies for managing these situations, as they are not uncommon. Although specifics vary, most healthcare institu-tions have policies in place requiring documentation by two physicians, the treating physician, and a consultant, that a decision needs to be made emergently in order to proceed with lifesaving interventions.

It is important to note that even in cases where patients may lack the capacity to make their own medical decisions (e.g., consenting for medication or planning disposition), they may still retain the capacity to appoint a surrogate healthcare proxy. Analogous to the capacity requirement for the health-care decision itself, in order to have capacity to appoint a surrogate decision-maker, a patient must demonstrate an awareness of the need to have a surrogate, the ability to iden-tify a choice of surrogate and to express a logical rationale for choosing that individual.

Performing a Capacity Assessment

Capacity is "not a scientifically determinable state and is situation specific [4]." The outcome of capacity assessments depends not only on the nature of the decision needing to be made, but also on the context in which the question arises. Not all capacity questions are created equal. Rather, a patient's decision-making capacity exists on a continuum. This capacity continuum comprises the relative risks and benefits of the choices available to the patient and the risks and benefits of the choice a patient purports to make. Understanding consequences to patients with regards to their autonomy and independent decision-making is para-mount for any provider completing a capacity assessment [5].

A thorough and thoughtful capacity evaluation requires balancing patient autonomy with other core ethical principles such as beneficence (maximizing patient benefit) and non-maleficence (do no harm) [5].

The greater the benefit and lower the risk of a purported choice, the less "capacitated"—the less sophisticated—a patient's understanding needs to be in order to accept that choice. Conversely, when the benefits of a purported choice are low and risks are high, patients must demonstrate a greater level of understanding in order to make a capacitated choice. It is for this reason that a patient presenting with severe substernal chest pain radiating to the left arm can easily make a capacitated decision to accept a cardiac workup but would be required to have a very well thought out rationale for leaving the hospital against medical advice. The benefits of a cardiac workup in this context are potentially lifesaving and the risks are relatively low (i.e., blood loss related to a needlestick, possible infection, etc.). The consequences of deciding to leave the hospital, however, are very different. The benefits of leaving are relatively few-avoiding needle sticks and chances of infection, saving money and/or insurance benefits, and avoiding the somewhat uncomfortable hassle of navigating the emergency medical system. The risks of leaving in this situation are exceedingly high, including the distinct possibility of death. Note, however, that a patient could, even in these circumstances, meet a capacity standard. For example, where he or she is able to explain that they have a terminal illness and are no longer interested in lifesaving interventions, or that they ascribe to a religion that does not accept medical care, they may be able to present a rational and clear case for their decision. It would be difficult, but not impossible, in these scenarios to meet the capacity requirement to make the decision to leave the hospital against medical advice.

To further illustrate how this continuum works, consider the following example from the perspective of the capacity to refuse a particular test, the complete blood count (CBC). A 78-year-old man is admitted to the hospital with diverticulitis.

After routine care, he demonstrates significant clinical improvement and his team feels confident he is ready for discharge. On the morning of scheduled discharge, he refuses his morning CBC. The threshold for this to be a capacitated decision is quite low. This conclusion stems from the fact that the benefits, re-confirming the patient is doing well, are relatively low. However, if this same 78-year-old man was in the acute phase of his illness and had a known history of gastrointestinal bleeding that had led to severe anemia and hypoxia, the benefits of knowing whether the patient's hemoglobin was critically low would be high and the risks low. To refuse blood work for laboratory testing in this scenario, the patient would need to demonstrate a clear understanding of the situation, including the relevant background of anemia and gastrointestinal bleeding, a well thought through rationale for refusing the CBC test, and a clear understanding of the consequences of his decision, including the possibility that he would die.

These examples demonstrate, as with any proposed intervention, refusing a CBC depends heavily on the context in which the decision arises. As the latter example also suggests, it is not uncommon that a patient has the capacity to make one choice, but not another.

In addition, capacity is not an all or nothing proposition. Incapacity for making one medical decision does not necessarily mean incapacity to make another or all decisions. For example, a 68-year-old woman with moderate dementia may not have the capacity to accept or refuse a necessary surgery, but she may retain the wherewithal to identify her spouse, child, or other family members as someone who knows her well and has always looked out for her. If she understands that she needs someone to serve as a surrogate and wants to appoint this person, she very likely has the requisite capacity to do so.

Finally, it is not altogether uncommon for patients to refuse to participate in a capacity assessment. Such refusals pose particular challenges to providers. First, it deprives the clinician of determining whether the patient accurately understands his or her medical condition(s) and options for care. Second, the patient's rationale for the purported decision may not be known. Hurst argues that a patient's refusal to convey a rationale for making a choice does not necessarily translate to incapacity [6]. It simply prevents the clinician from making a capacity determination. In such circumstances, Hurst advocates physicians engage their patients in further conversation or find an alternate provider with whom the patient may be more comfortable speaking [6]. If the patient continues refusing to have their capacity assessed, the risk of proceeding with a patient's wish should be weighed by their providers; if the risk is significantly high, clinicians should proceed as if the patient were incapacitated. If possible, this decision should be shared with the patient, and the patient informed that decision-making will be deferred to their surrogate.

Clinician Confidence in Performing Capacity Assessments

Academic literature reflects that clinicians are not altogether confident in performing capacity assessments [7]. One of the primary concerns among healthcare providers is the ability to detect incapacity in patients with cognitive impairment. A study by Sessums et al. showed that up to 40% of providers did not correctly identify incapacitated patients, raising the question: are we allowing incapacitated patients to make medical decisions? [4].

Clinicians lack of confidence is by no means specialty or location specific [7]. A recent study from New Zealand surveying various specialists' attitudes about performing capacity assessments found that only 28% of clinicians working in a hospital setting felt comfortable assessing a patient's capacity in most cases. Even fewer general practitioners (15%) felt comfortable making capacity assessments in most cases [7]. Providers identified several areas of concern, including time constraints, gaps in understanding the legal system, and difficulty with managing and accounting for the potential effects of comorbid psychiatric disorders.

These findings are consistent with previous results by Ganzini et al. suggesting that additional educational efforts at all levels of training are necessary to address key pitfalls in making capacity determinations [8].

Medical Decision-Making and the Elderly

Elderly patients are at high risk for becoming incapacitated. This may be due to a variety of causes, most notably dementia [9–11]. Other potential causes of incapacity among elderly patients include delirium, infections, neurological disorders, psychosis, mood disorders, substance abuse, sensory impairments, and medications (particularly those that are sedating) [11, 12]. Although these are risk factors for incapacity in any patient, elderly individuals tend to be more susceptible to these risk factors. Often times these risk factors for incapacity may occur concurrently in patients. Additionally, elderly patients may be at higher risk of having states of impairment go unrecognized [13]. While medical diagnoses alone, regardless of the degree of severity, are not sufficient for a determination of incapacity, it may inform evaluations and provide useful frameworks for conducting capacity assessments [14]. As much as possible, underlying contributors to a state of incapacity should be treated prior to declaring a patient incapacitated or pursuing aggressive measures such as court-appointed guardianship [9]. In patients with contributing sensory deficits such as hearing loss or visual impairment, modifying communication tools may be helpful. Clinicians should consider using aids such as pictures, illustrations, diagrams, or amplifiers [9]. If providers are assessing capacity in an inpatient setting, modifications may need to be made to the environment such as minimizing noise and distractions [9]. Providers should make their best effort to assess patients suffering from delirium when they are most lucid [11]. In short, when an elderly patient's capacity is called into question, every effort should be made to minimize any potential confounding factors. When a patient is considered incapacitated, they are being deprived of autonomy, which should not be taken lightly [5]. Additionally, providers should obtain collateral information about a patient's pre-morbid functioning, prior healthcare decision-making, and values [14]. Potential sources of collateral information include other providers, family members, friends, neighbors, or others who may know the patient well.

Medical Decision-Making and Dementia

Patients with dementia are at high risk for losing medical decision-making capacity as their neurodegenerative disease progresses [13]. Cognitive deficits in patients with dementia may include worsening of one or more of the following areas: memory, attention, executive functions, visuospatial skills, and language. Deficits in one or all of these domains may impact a patient's medical decision-making ability. In a sample of elderly patients, the presence of cognitive impairment was strongly associated with a lack of decision-making capacity [10]. However, medical decision-making ability is not the same thing as cognitive ability [11]. Patients may retain medical decision-making early on in their disease process, despite the presence of cognitive deficits. Additionally, many dementia spectrum illnesses are associated with fluctuating cognition; this may occur most frequently in dementia with Lewy bodies, but has also been noted in Alzheimer's disease, Parkinson's disease, and vascular dementia [9].

As dementias are progressive illnesses, capacity should be frequently re-assessed among individuals with dementia [12]. Involving family and caregivers in decision-making when patients still retain capacity may help ease future conflicts when surrogate decision-makers are necessary [15, 16]. Patients with dementia should be allowed to participate in medical decision-making to the extent that they are able, even if they have been declared incompetent [11]. A declaration of incompetency should not negate the patient's preferences or desires [5]. Clinicians may help mitigate confusion caused by cognitive deficits by using simple and easily comprehensible language in their discussions [9]. If feasible, providers should have conversations with patients about a specific medical decision more than once. Although patients may lose orientation to time and place, if there is consistency in their response regarding a specific medical concern, this may give providers and potential surrogate decision-makers insight into their underlying preferences, values, and core beliefs [11]. As patients with dementia typically have greater difficulty with the understanding and reasoning aspects of the four central tenants of medical decision-making capacity, providers may want to pay particular attention to these two aspects of a capacity assessment [17].

Once a surrogate decision-maker has been appointed, there are two broad approaches to decision-making [5]. In the substituted judgment standard, surrogates base decisions on what they believe the patient would have decided had they been able to do so [5, 12, 15, 16]. This may be difficult for surrogates who lack prior knowledge of a patient's goals or wishes (as may be the case with a court-appointed surrogates or non-family members) [15, 16]. Even in cases where the surrogate knows the patient well, lack of prior conversations about important healthcare decision points such as end-of-life care, are often cited as barriers [15, 16]. In the best interest standard, surrogates base decisions on what would be in the patient's current best interest, taking into consideration items such as degree of suffering, current and prior functioning, and quality of life [5, 15, 16]. Both types of decision-making should take into account the patient's values and goals to the greatest extent possible [5]. Surrogate decision-makers may want to involve other family or close friends in the decision-making process; however, while this may help clarify a patient's underlying wishes, it can alternatively lead to discord and greater uncertainty [15, 16].

When patients have known degenerative disorders such as dementia that have a high likelihood of leading to incapacity, providers should consider initiating conversations about treatment preferences early on in the disease process [15, 16]. Encouraging patients to think about what type of care they may wish to receive in the late stages of their disease may help them articulate these wishes to future surrogate decision-makers. While documents such as living wills may make some specifications about interventions, particularly at the end of life, they are generally unable to anticipate every potential medical scenario. In these instances, if patients and their families have had robust discussions about core beliefs related to medical care, surrogates may feel more confident that they are making decisions consistent with the patient's desires [5, 12, 15, 16].

The Role of Standardized Cognitive Assessments and Capacity Assessment Tools

Common tools for assessing cognition include the Folstein Mini-Mental Status Examination (MMSE), the Montreal Cognitive Assessment (MOCA), the St. Louis University Mental Status (SLUMS), and the Mini-Cog, although numerous other tools exist in clinical practice and research settings [17]. Providers should be aware that while these tests assess a variety of cognitive domains, they may be insensitive to mild cognitive impairment [13]. A patient's score on any of these tests alone does not determine their ability to make a medical decision. Each of these standardized cognitive tests is a potential aid rather than a substitute for a comprehensive capacity evaluation [11]. In some cases, full neuropsychological batteries may be helpful [14]. Research suggests that in patients with known dementia, impairments in naming, delayed memory, and inflexibility on cognitive testing may be the best predictors of incapacity [18]. Understanding which cognitive domains are significantly impaired in a particular patient may also help clinicians tailor conversations about medical decisions in such a way as to maximize the patient's ability to comprehend and participate in the assessment process.

Several tools have been developed to identify incapacity and better standardize capacity assessments. Although a clinical interview remains the standard of care for performing a capacity assessment, limitations in the provider's scope of practice and clinical discomfort with performing capacity assessments can affect the validity of the result. One of the most validated tools for capacity assessments is the MacArthur competence assessment tool-treatment (MacCAT-T), a semi-structured interview tool that assesses the previously described four domains of capacity [19]. A score is assigned at the conclusion of the assessment, signifying the quality of answers to questions in the four domains. The tool has high inter-rater reliability and has particular utility in difficult cases, or when providers disagree on clinical examination alone [19]. Finally, the MacCAT-T is highly recommended for clinicians who do not regularly make capacity determinations for older adults [20].

Additional tools for assessing capacity include the assessment of capacity for everyday decision-making (ACED), aid to capacity evaluation (ACE), Hopemont capacity assessment interview (HCAI), and the capacity to consent to treatment instrument (CCTI) [21–24]. The ACED is a semi-structured interview, similar to the MacCAT-T; however, its developers posit this tool is superior to the MacCAT-T for patients with mild to moderate dementia, especially in cases where clinicians are concerned for self-neglect [21]. A more simplistic tool is the ACE, which allows clinicians to document observations in a methodical way to better synthesize data from their clinical interview. Most importantly, this tool also ensures depression and psychosis are ruled out before making a capacity determination. The HCAI and CCTI utilize hypothetical vignettes to assess reasoning, understanding, and appreciation. In a direct comparison between the HCAI, CCTI, and MacCAT-T, there was notably poor agreement in findings between these tools [25].

Finally, the University of California, San Diego Brief Assessment of Capacity to Consent (UBACC) was developed as a screening tool to identify cases that may need further investigation to make a determination of capacity. This 10-question screen takes 5 minutes or less to administer and may be particularly germane in research settings [26].

Conclusions

Determining medical decision-making capacity is a clinical judgment made by physicians. This is in contrast to competency, which is a legal term. In order to have capacity, patients are typically required to exhibit four key features: a basic understanding of the medical issues at play, appreciation of the risks and benefits, communication a choice, and the ability to communicate the rationale for their decision. It is important for clinicians to structure clinical interviews around these four components of capacitated decision-making in addition to considering the severity and medical implications of the situation at hand. In elderly patients, cognitive impairment, due to delirium, dementia, or both, may make clinical assessments of capacity more complicated. Clinicians providing long-term care to patients with a known neurodegenerative disorder should consider initiating conversations about medical decision-making with patients early in their disease process. Standardized assessments of capacity and screening tools for cognitive impairment may provide useful aids for clinicians faced with these scenarios.

References

1. Appelbaum P, Grisso T. Assessing patients' capacities to consent to treatment. NEJM. 1988;319(25):1635–8.
2. Appelbaum P. Assessment of patients' competence to consent to treatment. NEJM. 2007;357(18):1834–40.
3. Farrell TW, Widera E, Rosenberg L, Rubin CD, Naik AD, Braun U, et al. AGS position statement: making medical treatment decisions for unbefriended older adults. J Am Geriatr Soc. 2016;65(1):14–5.

4. Sessums LL, Zembrzuska H, Jackson JL. Does this patient have medical decision-making capacity? JAMA. 2011;306(4):420.
5. Boyle R. Determining patients' capacity to share in decision-making. In: Fletcher JC, Spencer EM, Lombardo PA, editors. Fletcher's introduction to clinical ethics. 3rd ed. Hagerstown: University Publishing Group; 2005. p. 117–38.
6. Hurst SA. When patients refuse assessment of decision-making capacity. Arch Intern Med. 2004;164(16):1757.
7. Young G, Douglass A, Davison L. What do doctors know about assessing decision-making capacity? N Z Med J. 2018;131(1471):58–71.
8. Ganzini L, Volicer L, Nelson W, Derse A. Pitfalls in assessment of decision-making capacity. Psychosomatics. 2003;44(3):237–43.
9. Trachsel M, Hermann H, Biller-Andorno N. Cognitive fluctuations as a challenge for the assessment of decision-making capacity in patients with dementia. Am J Alzheimers Dis Other Demen. 2015;30(4):360–3.
10. Boettger S, Bergman M, Jenewin J, Boettger S. Advanced age and decisional capacity: the effect of age on the ability to make health care decisions. Arch Gerontol Geriatr. 2016;66:211–7.
11. Ganzini L, Volicer L, Nelson W, Fox E, Derse AR. Ten myths about decision-making capacity. J Am Med Dir Assoc. 2004;5(3 Suppl):263–7.
12. Rodin M, Mohile S. Assessing decisional capacity in the elderly. Semin Oncol. 2008;35(6):625–32.
13. Edersheim J, Murray E, Padmanabhan J, Price BH. Protecting the health and finances of the elderly with early cognitive impairment. J Am Acad Psychiatry Law. 2017;45(1):81–91.
14. Falk E, Hoffman N. The role of capacity assessments in elder abuse investigations and guardianship. Clin Geriatr Med. 2014;30(4):851–68.
15. Fetherstonhaugh D, McAuliffe L, Bauer M, Shanley C. Decision-making on behalf of people living with dementia: how do surrogate decision-makers decide? J Med Ethics. 2017;43(1):35–40.
16. Fetherstonhaugh D, McAuliffe L, Shanley C, Bauer M, Beattie E. "Did I make the right decision?": the difficult journey of being a surrogate decision maker for a person living with dementia. Dementia (London). 2017;0:1–14.
17. Lin JS, O'Connor E, Rossom R, Perdue LA, Burda BU, Thompson M, et al. Screening for cognitive impairment in older adults: an evidence update for the U.S. Preventive Services Task Force. Evid Synth. 2013;107:1–403.

18. Moye J, Karel M, Gurrera R, Azar AR. Neuropsychological predictors of decision-making capacity over 9 months in mild-to-moderate dementia. J Gen Intern Med. 2006;21(1):78–83.
19. Grisso T, Appelbaum PS, Hill-Fotouhi C. The MacCAT-T: a clinical tool to assess patients' capacities to make treatment decisions. Psychiatr Serv. 1997;48(11):1415–9.
20. Porrino P, Falcone Y, Agosta L, Isaia G, Zanocchi M, Mastrapasqua A, et al. Informed consent in older medical inpatients: assessment of decision-making capacity. J Am Geriatr Soc. 2015;63(11):2423–4.
21. Lai JM, Gill TM, Cooney LM, Bradley EH, Hawkins KA, Karlawish JH. Everyday decision-making ability in older persons with cognitive impairment. Am J Geriatr Psychiatry. 2008;16(8):693–6.
22. Baird AD, Solcz SL, Gale-Ross R, Blake TM. Older adults and capacity-related assessment: promise and caution. Exp Aging Res. 2009;35(3):297–316.
23. Etchells E, Darzins P, Silberfeld M, Singer PA, Mckenny J, Naglie G. Assessment of patient capacity to consent to treatment. J Gen Intern Med. 1999;14(1):27–34.
24. Gerstenecker A, Niccolai L, Marson D, Triebel KL. Enhancing medical decision-making evaluations: introduction of normative data for the capacity to consent to treatment instrument. Assessment. 2016;23(2):232–9.
25. Gurrera RJ, Karel MJ, Azar AR, Moye J. Agreement between instruments for rating treatment decisional capacity. Am J Geriatr Psychiatry. 2007;15(2):168–73.
26. Jeste DV, Palmer BW, Appelbaum PS, Golshan S, Glorioso D, Dunn LB, et al. A new brief instrument for assessing decisional capacity for clinical research. Arch Gen Psychiatry. 2007;64(8):966.

Chapter 3
The Capacity to Live Independently

Mary E. Camp and Alexander Cole

Introduction

As stated by Cooney et al., "The freedom to live where and as one chooses is one of the most basic of human rights" [1], and the decision to remove someone from their home against their will cannot be taken lightly. In some cases, the transition to a supported and structured living environment is a clear need, based on immediate and serious safety concerns in the setting of a person with an inability to understand and appreciate the risks of their living environment. However, in many cases, the decision-making process surrounding independent living is less clear cut. The decision to live independently is a multifaceted issue, involving personal preference, cultural norms, finances, health, safety, social support, among other factors.

The complexity of this process is reflected in several large studies examining the factors associated with nursing home placement. In a meta-analysis involving 178,056 individuals 65 or older, Gaugler et al. found a heterogeneous list of factors associated with admission to a nursing home: cognitive impairment, three or more Activity of Daily Living (ADL)

M. E. Camp (✉) · A. Cole
University of Texas Southwestern Medical Center, Dallas, TX, USA
e-mail: Molly.Camp@UTSouthwestern.edu;
Alexander.Cole@phhs.org

© Springer Nature Switzerland AG 2019   37
M. Balasubramaniam et al. (eds.), *Psychiatric Ethics in Late-Life Patients*, https://doi.org/10.1007/978-3-030-15172-0_3

dependencies, Caucasian race/ethnicity, male gender, lack of a spouse, fewer living children, not owning ones' own home, recent hospitalization, prior nursing home admission, lower annual income, increased age, history of falls, or specific health conditions (diabetes, hypertension, cancer, or stroke) [2].

In a systematic review, Luppa et al. found strong evidence for the following predisposing factors for nursing home admission: increased age, not owning one's own house, Caucasian (if American), low self-rated health status, functional impairment in ADL and instrumental ADL (IADL), cognitive impairment, dementia diagnosis, prior nursing home placement, and higher number of prescriptions [3]. Moderate to weak evidence was found for being unmarried, unemployed, and having a poor social network.

Dementia is often quoted as the number one cause of institutionalization in older adults [4]. Luppa et al. found that 20% of seniors (65 years of older) moved to institutionalized living in the first year of diagnosis of dementia, and that this rate increased to 50% by 5 years after diagnosis [3]. The median time to institutionalization was 30–40 months. Rates of institutionalization were higher in individuals with greater age, lower levels of education, Caucasian ethnicity (compared to African American or Hispanic individuals in particular), more severe cognitive deficits, greater functional impairment, and behavioral and psychological symptoms of dementia. Rates were also greater for those who were unmarried or living alone. The desire to move to institutionalized living also decreased the time for this to happen.

In addition, caregiver attributes impacted the rates of institutionalization. Those individuals with caregivers who were relatives but not spouses experienced higher rates of institutionalization [4]. Rates also increased if the caregiver experienced higher levels of caregiver burden, lower perceived quality of life, or fewer supportive social contacts. Rates increased if the caregiver was employed, had a higher salary, or higher level of education. Increased in-home help decreased institutionalization.

Therefore, the decision whether or not to transition to a supported living environment goes beyond personal preference. Additionally, safety factors (i.e., whether the individual can safely maintain their own living environment) and other psychosocial determinants including finances and caregiver attributes also play a role. Although dementia is not the only reason why an older person may need a more supported living environment, it a common reason, and while many people with dementia retain decisional capacity, the presence of a cognitive disorder may complicate the process of making this determination [5].

In this chapter, we will review the literature on conceptualizations, frameworks, and specific methods for assessing a person's capacity for independent living.

Risks and Benefits of Institutionalization

Risks and benefits of a transition to structured or supervised living environment will depend on characteristics of the individual and his or her psychosocial circumstances. It would be impossible to describe all of the potential contributors related to culture, finances, availability of housing, medical contributors, and family influences that one may face in making this assessment. However, some relevant literature can provide some over-arching findings related to older adults' views of institutional living compared to aging in place in the community.

In a meta-synthesis of 128 individuals in 24 nursing homes, Vaismoradi et al. reported that the most common reason for transition to nursing home was that the person and/or family were unable to meet the person's needs in the community [6]. Accordingly, the benefit of nursing home was in "being taken care of" in an environment of cleanliness, safety, and professional/respectful interactions with nursing staff. Others reported a sense of "relief and security" when they were no longer responsible for activities of daily living at home [7].

In a study of 3262 medically ill older adults with increased care needs, only 7% of the individuals said that they were "very willing" to live permanently in a nursing home, while 30% said that they would "rather die." Notably, surrogates only reported the exact understanding of the older adults' preference in 37% of cases [8]. While individuals will certainly have a variety of personal preference on the topic, for some, staying at home is preferable to a nursing home, even at the risk of harm to self.

Proponents of aging in place (referring to living with some level of independence in the community) believe that aging in place may allow an individual to experience independence, autonomy, attachment, connection, and security related to being in a familiar place [9]. Some literature on older adults' perceptions of nursing home life reports that organizational constraints may lead to residents feeling "hurried," "controlled" due to lack of flexibility, and even "helpless." Furthermore, the residents in question reported that the nursing homes themselves, due to the inherent constraints of institutionalized living, resulted in restricted decision-making in general. Other studies have indicated that the perception of life control impacts the nursing home residents' sense of dignity [10] and that the qualities of the nursing home organization and staff may promote or limit residents' actualization of their own free will [11]. Furthermore, leaving one's home and transitioning to a new environment may result in feelings of loss or stress [7].

The determination of capacity does not hinge on the examiner's appraisal of the risks and benefits of nursing home placement but, rather, on the individual's ability to understand and reason through their own individual risks and benefits, as will be discussed in the following section.

Assessment of Capacity to Live Independently

When considering whether an individual has the capacity to care for oneself, Naik et al. recommend evaluating five domains of safe and independent living [12]:

1. Personal needs and hygiene: This domain includes basic self-care activities such as bathing, dressing, and toileting. Ambulation, transfer ability, and associated fall risk may also be considered in this domain.

2. The condition of the home environment: This domain includes basic maintenance and repairs of the home, including access to electricity and water, a sufficiently sanitary living environment, and avoidance of other safety hazards (fire, structural deficiencies of the home, etc.).

3. Activities for independent living: This domain evaluates whether the person can complete complex tasks at home, including shopping, meal preparation, cleaning, transportation, and using technology.

4. Medical self-care: This domain encompasses medication management, wound care, and appropriate illness self-monitoring.

5. Financial affairs and estate: This domain gauges the person's ability to pay bills on time, track his or her finances, avoid exploitation, and enter into binding contracts when needed.

An individual does not need to be able to independently complete all of these tasks to live independently. Assistance from home visitation programs may prolong a person's ability to live at home with assistance [13], but the person would need to acknowledge the need for, or at least accept the help from, these services. These five domains should be evaluated in a variety of ways during a comprehensive assessment to assess an older adult's ability to live independently.

The capacity to live independently presents unique challenges because it involves not only a person's ability to make a decision about their wishes, but also their ability to carry out tasks associated with those wishes [14]. Unlike consent to certain forms of medical treatment in which someone else administers the treatment, the person who chooses to live at home will then have responsibility for caring for him or herself or recruiting/allowing help in areas where assistance is needed. For this reason, the capacity for independent living may be evaluated using the "articulate →demonstrate" method [15]. That is, the person should be asked to articulate decisional capacity and demonstrate executive capacity.

Decisional Capacity

Details about capacity assessment in older adults will be covered elsewhere in this book, but in this chapter, we will adapt Grisso and Appelbaum's MacArthur Competence Assessment Tool for Treatment to evaluate capacity for independent living [16]:

1. *Understanding:* This involves the individual's ability to recall factual content related to the situation and describe a fairly clear version of it (preferably paraphrased, not recited verbatim from the examiner). This information should include associated risks and benefits, as well as a reasonably accurate indication of the likelihood of each choice. In this case, the person will need to understand what demands are being placed on him or her due to independent living status, and the risks of being unable to manage those demands.
2. *Appreciation:* The person acknowledges that the situation at hand applies to him or her directly, and that the information presented is manifesting in his or her life.
3. *Reasoning:* The person is able to list specific consequences of his or her choice, including how these consequences will impact their everyday life. The person can compare at least two options and identify differences between them. The final choice should follow from the person's own reasoning as articulated in their explanations.
4. *Expressing a choice:* The person states a clear and consistent choice for a preferred solution or course of action. In more advanced cases of dementia, individuals may have difficulty verbalizing a consistent choice, but this ability is likely to be preserved in more cognitively intact individuals [14]. However, in the authors' clinical experience, changes in external factors (finances or health needs) may cause a person to change from a previously longstanding stated preference, which may surprise or complicate the situation for surrogate decision-makers.

Executive Capacity

Even if a person expresses verbal decisional capacity, it does not guarantee that he or she will be able to dutifully perform the assigned tasks. For the individual to complete one's decisions, they must have what is called as the "*executive capacity*." Executive capacity requires that a person be able to formulate a plan, modify the plan in case of unexpected changes, and delegate responsibilities to surrogates when needed [12]. In evaluating executive capacity, clinicians can draw on a variety of sources of information to evaluate past, present, and future performance [15].

First, it may be important to consider past performance. For instance, if someone is able to describe the appropriate steps in adhering to his or her diabetes regimen but their hemoglobin A1c indicates poor glucose control over the past 3 months, this may be an indication of impaired executive capacity.

Present performance will also bear relevance to executive capacity. This can be evaluated by examining the person's present state when compared to their stated goals of self-care. For instance, the evaluator may consider whether the person has adequate hygiene, maintains a healthy weight, and attends appointments as scheduled. Cognitive and functional assessments (described below) may help evaluate executive capacity. Home visits by the treatment team are also extremely helpful, if available to further evaluate the safety of the home environment. In cases where this is a concern for serious or dangerous self-neglect, social services may also become involved for a home safety evaluation.

While future performance typically cannot be guaranteed, diagnoses such as dementia that is likely to progress would need to be considered in longer term planning. Similarly, if the person has a physical injury that is likely to improve, this may also warrant consideration.

As noted above, capacity to live independently does not hinge on the person's ability to perform all activities of daily living independently, but to be able to understand the need for assistance if present, and to delegate appropriately to maintain one's safety.

Cognitive Assessment

Before discussing specific measures of cognitive assessment, it is important to note that no single cognitive assessment tool is capable of definitively assessing an individual's capacity to live independently, even if an assessment reveals evidence for significant cognitive impairment. Formal cognitive assessments are an important, but not a definitive component of the independent living assessment. Often the individual's performance on cognitive assessments only weakly predicts their ability to perform activities of daily living especially in mild cognitive impairment [17]. As the degree of cognitive impairment becomes more severe, poor performance on cognitive assessments is more strongly associated with functional decline [18]. These limitations in formal cognitive assessments highlight the importance of a thorough, patient-centered assessment which includes, but is not based solely on, a formal cognitive assessment.

A variety of cognitive assessments have been developed and are available for clinical use. Some assessments, such as the Folstein Mini-Mental State Examination (F-MMSE), the Montreal Cognitive Assessment (MoCA), Addenbrooke's Cognitive Examination (ACE), and the Short Portable Mental Status Questionnaire (SPMSQ), aim to quickly provide a global assessment of an individual's cognitive ability by briefly assessing a variety of cognitive domains. The specific domains assessed vary among individual instruments, but typically they include tests of memory, orientation, and attention. Tests of executive functioning and visuospatial skills may also be included. Other assessments like the Wisconsin Card Sorting Test (WCST), the animal naming test (ANT), and the Visual Object and Space Perception Test thoroughly evaluate single cognitive domains.

As noted above, global cognitive assessments have been shown to have little value as stand-alone functional and capacity assessments, particularly when only minimal cognitive impairment is present. Among individuals with mild cognitive impairment as determined by global cognitive assessments,

ADLs remain preserved and are often equivalent to those without cognitive impairment [19]. Furthermore, an individual's level of education is positively associated with performance on global cognitive assessment, complicating the interpretation of results. While more severe cognitive impairment identified on these assessments is associated with poor functional performance, assessment of global cognitive functioning alone is not sufficient to assess functional ability. The primary value of global assessments of cognition may instead lie in longitudinal assessments, thus allowing the clinician to track a patient's course over time and provide prognostic information about their course and potential care needs in the future rather than assessing an individual's overall functional status at present [20].

Clinicians should also recognize that all global cognitive assessments are not created equal. The F-MMSE for example is insensitive to mild cognitive impairment, whereas the SPMSQ is insensitive to small changes in cognitive ability [20]. Reviewing the performance characteristics of individual instruments is beyond the scope of this text, but the selection of a specific global assessment instrument should include consideration of the purpose of the assessment (e.g., one-time assessment versus longitudinal assessment), the expected severity of cognitive decline, the resources available to the clinician (e.g., the amount of time available to complete an assessment and the ability to pay for assessments, if necessary), and the availability of third-party informants (which is necessary to complete, for example in the Dementia Rating Scale).

Additional studies investigating the role of specific cognitive domains and the ability to function independently have revealed that executive functioning is strongly predictive of IADL performance, while memory and visuospatial performance also play critical roles in the maintenance of IADLs [21]. Assessment of individual cognitive domains may reveal impairments that are not identified on global cognitive assessments and allow the clinician to better characterize deficits and guide treatment recommendations, particularly with respect to the decision of where an individual should live and what types of assistance may be necessary for them to live safely. As with global cognitive assessments, a thorough review of the assessments available and characteristics of individual instruments is outside the scope of this text. Detailed testing of specific cognitive domains may be indicated when global cognitive function is found to be intact, but a person or caregiver describes a clear decline in day-to-day functioning.

Functional Assessment

As with cognitive assessments, numerous functional assessment instruments have been developed and are used in clinical practice [22]. Functional assessment instruments are not intended to provide the clinician with a dichotomous, "yes/no" recommendation for a person's ability to live independently; instead, they attempt to objectively assess how well a person can perform a variety of tasks critical to self-management and self-care. The clinician then uses the results of these assessments along with other factors unique to an individual's presentation to guide their recommendation for the individual to live independently or if necessary the extent and types of assistance that may be necessary to allow the individual to live safely in the community.

Some assessments focus on particular skill domains—for example, the Medication Management Ability Assessment (MMAA), the Financial Capacity Index (FCI), and the Kitchen Task Assessment (KTA)—while others (e.g., the Cognitive Performance Test) assess multiple domains and attempt to provide a broad assessment of a person's ability to successfully perform ADLs and IADLs [22]. Individual assessments vary widely, with some capable of being administered quickly in the clinic setting and others requiring extensive materials and/or administration at home [23]. The time required to complete an individual assessment also varies significantly: brief assessments (e.g., the ADL Situational Test) may take as little as 15 minutes, while more extensive assessments (e.g., the Refined ADL Assessment Scale) may take 90 minutes or more [22]. Specific skills assessed on functional assessments include operating a telephone, maintaining hygiene, independently managing finances, taking medications correctly, safely preparing and eating meals, and other skills, often by direct observation with a clinician. Individual assessments vary in the sets of skills assessed [23].

Moore et al. performed a systematic review of more than 30 functional assessments described in the literature with the goal of identifying instruments most suitable for use in a clinical setting [22]. For individuals with a known neurocognitive disorder, the Cognitive Performance Test (CPT), Direct Assessment of Functional Status (DAFS), Structured Assessment of Independent Living Skills (SAILS), Occupational Therapy Evaluation of Performance and Support (OTEPS), and the Occupational Therapy Assessment Scale (OTAS) are recommended for functional assessment. The Everyday Problems Test (EPT), Independent Living Scales (ILS), and Observed Tasks of Daily Living (OTDL) assessments are recommended in otherwise healthy older individuals, while the ILS and UCSD Performance-Based Skills Assessment (USPA) are recommended in individuals with serious mental illness [22]. These assessments were generally found to be internally consistent, have high interrater and retest reliability, and correlate well with more extensive methods to evaluate daily functioning.

Framework of Evaluation

Clearly, assessing all of these domains requires a great deal of time and interdisciplinary involvement. Skelton et al. describe the "Capacity Assessment and Intervention" (CAI) model developed at the Baylor College of Medicine in Houston [15]. This model involves an interdisciplinary team of geriatricians, social workers, a nurse case manager, occupational therapists, and physical therapists who complete a thorough cognitive, medical, and functional assessment. In doing so, the team visits the patient's home and involves family members as well as social services if needed. The team also completes a 6-month follow-up to reassess capacity and help the patient move toward individualized goals. A thorough functional assessment and implementation of a plan based on associated findings requires a great deal of time and energy and involves multiple providers. Ideally, this would happen in the context of an interdisciplinary team, as in the CAI model. However, in many contexts, this may require the involvement of practitioners from different disciplines across separate systems with a focus on communication across disciplines.

Implications of Incapacity to Decide to Live at Home

Although the full legal ramifications of this sort of capacity evaluation are outside of the scope of this chapter, it is worth noting that the assessment of capacity may lead to findings that will require legal intervention to ensure the safety of the person in question [24]. In these cases, the practitioner would need to consider the following: (1) Which specific tasks the person can and cannot do; (2) What decisions the person can or cannot make; (3) What are the risks of not intervening; and (4) How far an intervention should go to help the person [1]. Even if a person does not have the capacity to decide whether to live independently, surrogate decision-makers may not necessarily choose institutionalization. Rather, they can work toward finding the least restrictive living environment that is closest to the person's prior stated wishes but also provides adequate safety provisions.

Conclusion

Determination of capacity to live independently involves a multifaceted and interdisciplinary approach to evaluate decisional and executive capacity in the five domains of safe and independent living. The exact risks and benefits will vary from person to person, involving a myriad of factors from personal preference to changing realities of financial and medical needs.

References

1. Cooney LM, Kennedy GJ, Hawkins KA, Hurme SB. Who can stay at home? Assessing the capacity to choose to live in the community. Arch Intern Med. 2004;164(4):357–60. https://doi.org/10.1001/archinte.164.4.357.
2. Gaugler JE, Duval S, Anderson KA, Kane RL. Predicting nursing home admission in the U.S: a meta-analysis. BMC Geriatr. 2007;7:13. https://doi.org/10.1186/1471-2318-7-13.
3. Luppa M, Luck T, Brahler E, Konig HH, Riedel-Heller SG. Prediction of institutionalisation in dementia. A systematic review. Dement Geriatr Cogn Disord. 2008;26(1):65–78. https://doi.org/10.1159/000144027.
4. Aguero-Torres H, von Strauss E, Viitanen M, Winblad B, Fratiglioni L. Institutionalization in the elderly: the role of chronic diseases and dementia. Cross-sectional and longitudinal data from a population-based study. J Clin Epidemiol. 2001;54(8):795–801. https://doi.org/10.1016/S0895-4356(00)00371-1.
5. Kim SY, Karlawish JH, Caine ED. Current state of research on decision-making competence of cognitively impaired elderly persons. Am J Geriatr Psychiatry. 2002;10(2):151–65. https://doi.org/10.1097/00019442-200203000-00006.
6. Waismoradi M, Wang IL, Turunen H, Bondas T. Older people's experiences of care in nursing homes: a meta-synthesis. Int Nurs Rev. 2016;63(1):111–21. https://doi.org/10.1111/inr.12232.
7. Lee DT, Woo J, Mackenzie AE. A review of older people's experiences with residential care placement. J Adv Nurs. 2002;37(1):19–27. https://doi.org/10.1046/j.1365-2648.2002.02060.x.
8. Mattimore TJ, Wenger NS, Desbiens NA, Teno JM, Hamel MB, Liu H, et al. Surrogate and physician understanding of patients' preferences for living permanently in a nursing home. J Am Geriatr Soc. 1997;45(7):818–24. https://doi.org/10.1111/j.1532-5415.1997.tb01508.x.
9. Wiles JL, Leibing A, Guberman N, Reeve J, Allen RE. The meaning of "aging in place" to older people. Gerontologist. 2012;52(3):357–66. https://doi.org/10.1093/geront/gnr098.

10. Oosterveld-Vlug MG, Pasman HR, van Gennip IE, Muller MT, Willems DL, Onwuteaka-Philipsen BD. Dignity and the factors that influence it according to nursing home residents: a qualitative interview study. J Adv Nurs. 2014;70(1):97–106. https://doi.org/10.1111/jan.12171.

11. Tuominen L, Leino-Kilpi H, Suhonen R. Older people's experiences of their free will in nursing homes. Nurs Ethics. 2016;23(1):22–35. https://doi.org/10.1177/0969733014557119.

12. Naik AD, Lai JM, Kunik ME, Dyer CB. Assessing capacity in suspected cases of self-neglect. Geriatrics. 2008;63(2):24–31.

13. Stuck AE, Egger M, Hammer A, Minder CE, Beck JC. Home visits to prevent nursing home admission and functional decline in elderly people: systematic review and meta-regression analysis. JAMA. 2002;287(8):1022–8. https://doi.org/10.1001/jama.287.8.1022.

14. Lai JM, Karlawish J. Assessing the capacity to make everyday decisions: a guide for clinicians and an agenda for future research. Am J Geriatr Psychiatry. 2007;15(2):101–11. https://doi.org/10.1097/01.JGP.0000239246.10056.2e.

15. Skelton F, Kunik ME, Regev T, Naik AD. Determining if an older adult can make and execute decisions to live safely at home: a capacity assessment and intervention model. Arch Gerontol Geriatr. 2010;50(3):300–5. https://doi.org/10.1016/j.archger.2009.04.016.

16. Grisso T, Appelbaum PS. MacArthur competence assessment tool for treatment (MacCAT-T). Sarasota: Professional Resource Press; 1998.

17. Hill RD, Backman L, Fratiglioni L. Determinants of functional abilities in dementia. J Am Geriatr Soc. 1995;43(10):1092–7. https://doi.org/10.1111/j.1532-5415.1995.tb07006.x.

18. Njegovan V, Hing MM, Mitchell SL, Molnar FJ. The hierarchy of functional loss associated with cognitive decline in older persons. J Gerontol A Biol Sci Med Sci. 2001;56(10):M638–43. https://doi.org/10.1093/gerona/56.10.M638.

19. Jefferson AL, Byerly LK, Vanderhill S, Lambe S, Wong S, Ozonoff A, et al. Characterization of activities of daily living in individuals with mild cognitive impairment. Am J Geriatr Psychiatry. 2008;16(5):375–83. https://doi.org/10.1097/JGP.0b013e318162f197.

20. Applegate WB, Blass JP, Williams TF. Instruments for the functional assessment of older patients. N Engl J Med. 1990;322(17):1207–14. https://doi.org/10.1056/NEJM199004263221707.

21. Burton CL, Strauss E, Hultsch DF, Hunter MA. Cognitive functioning and everyday problem solving in older adults. Clin Neuropsychol. 2006;20(3):432–52. https://doi.org/10.1080/13854040590967063.

22. Moore DJ, Palmer BW, Patterson TL, Jeste DV. A review of performance-based measures of functional living skills. J Psychiatr Res. 2007;41(1–2):97–118. https://doi.org/10.1016/j.jpsychires.2005.10.008.

23. Desai AK, Grossberg GT, Sheth DN. Activities of daily living in patients with dementia: clinical relevance, methods of assessment and effects of treatment. CNS Drugs. 2014;18(13):853–75. https://doi.org/10.2165/00023210-200418130-00003.

24. Buchanan A. Mental capacity, legal competence, and consent to treatment. J R Soc Med. 2004;97(9):415–20. https://doi.org/10.1258/jrsm.97.9.415.

Chapter 4
The Capacity to Manage Finances

Oliver M. Glass, Larry Tune, and Adriana P. Hermida

Case Example

Ms. Smith is a 78-year-old Caucasian female who lives with her son in a home outside a metropolitan city. The son moved in three weeks ago after he called Ms. Smith informing him that he is homeless. An adult protective services (APS) report was filed by her daughter alleging that the son is taking Ms. Smith's money to buy opioid tablets off the streets. APS visits Ms. Smith's home and evaluates her alone. She is noticeably confused and is unaware of the current year or month. When asked to draw a clock, Ms. Smith drew a circle with all the hours in the top right-hand corner. She stated that she cannot remember who she banks with, but that her "son should know." When the son is interviewed by APS, he tells them that he is helping Ms. Smith with her bills and check writing

O. M. Glass (✉) · L. Tune · A. P. Hermida
Emory University, Department of Psychiatry and Behavioral Sciences, Atlanta, GA, USA
e-mail: oliver.glass@emory.edu; ltune@emory.edu; ahermid@emory.edu

© Springer Nature Switzerland AG 2019
M. Balasubramaniam et al. (eds.), *Psychiatric Ethics in Late-Life Patients*, https://doi.org/10.1007/978-3-030-15172-0_4

as she is "too confused" to do it on her own. The son then explained that he "just writes the checks and mom just signs them." He has slurred speech and is very restless during the evaluation. APS makes a referral for Ms. Smith to have a formal financial capacity assessment.

Introduction

In the coming years, clinicians are likely to be asked to provide expert opinion on whether patients have the capacity to manage their own finances. There will be increased demand, caused by (1) an aging population, (2) an increased prevalence of dementia, (3) a growth in per capita wealth, and (4) a higher frequency in divorce and remarriage [1]. A 2013 estimate found that at least 34% of the nation's wealth comes from older adults [2]. To add to this, a lack of financial capacity is directly correlated with financial exploitation. Dementia progresses slowly, where an exact demarcation of when someone loses their ability to manage their finances is hard to determine. Delirium, which may occur independently or with co-occurring dementia, typically has a waxing and waning of cognitive ability. Therefore, when someone is delirious, there may be lucid intervals where one may argue that the individual has capacity, but moments later, the person's consciousness may deteriorate. Evaluating monetary decision-making capacity can prove useful as it can be used to gauge whether one is at significant risk for financial exploitation. Individuals with dementia are especially vulnerable when it comes to financial exploitation, as they may lose twice as much money per case of financial exploitation when compared to those without a major neurocognitive disorder [3]. In this chapter, we will explore the relationship between aging and financial decision-making, while demonstrating how cognitive impairment may influence financial and testamentary capacity.

Financial and Testamentary Capacity

Financial Capacity

Mild cognitive impairment (MCI) and Alzheimer's dementia (AD) are often associated with lack of awareness of cognitive deficits [4, 5]. This impacts the individual's ability to pass the standard capacity assessment [6]. As a result, in the individual whose financial capacity is called into question, cognitive status must first be evaluated through a standardized screening tool. If necessary, financial capacity may need to be checked through neuropsychological testing. To make matters more complex, MCI and dementia are often associated with depression and apathy [7]. This can prove detrimental to an individual's ability to demonstrate capacity. Bayard et al. found that [8] those with MCI and AD are more likely to make disadvantageous selections on the Iowa Gambling Task (IGT). They are more likely to make choices that provide a high immediate reward despite the heightened risk for future punishment. Furthermore, the study found that individuals with MCI and AD performed similarly on the IGT [8]. Some people with MCI may develop disinhibition along with a lack of concern [9]. Disinhibition along with a lack of concern will likely contribute to poor financial decisions and an increased risk of financial exploitation. A person with isolated fronto-temporal impairments may in certain cases be able to conduct complex financial decisions but exhibit irrational behavior secondary to pathological impulsivity. Brain imaging combined with objective cognitive testing can be valuable when evaluating an individual for financial capacity.

Stoeckel et al. [10] found a relationship between atrophy of the medial frontal cortex in individuals with mild AD and poor performance on the Financial Capacity Instrument (FCI), indicating impairment in financial skills. The prefrontal cortex is particularly important in executive functioning [11]. Executive functioning impairment is directly correlated to poor financial skills [12]. The larger the prefrontal cortex volume in healthy individuals, the better the executive functioning [11]. When there is an imaging study which shows atrophy of this specific brain region, providers should assess for deficits in financial management. Objective cognitive measurement tools that have an executive functioning component (e.g., the Montreal Cognitive Assessment [MOCA]) can provide objective data to supplement the evaluator's assessment.

Testamentary Capacity

Testamentary decision-making capacity is the act of executing a will, and this capacity relies on the "ability to understand relevant facts and an appreciation of the reasonably foreseeable consequences of taking specific actions regarding the formation of a will" [13]. Testamentary capacity can be called into question when the individual is alive or deceased. The more the will deviates from the natural heir of inheritance, the more the individual must demonstrate a higher level of decision-making ability. In evaluating testamentary capacity where the will deviates from the natural heir(s), the evaluator should assess if the person understands who the natural heir to the inheritance is and the ability to appropriately describe the events that have led to the decision. The evaluator should determine whether there was any correlation between abnormal behaviors (e.g., whether there was an emergence of cognitive impairment) and the decision relating to the will. Shulman et al. [13] emphasized that the testator should demonstrate understanding of the following concepts when being evaluated for testamentary capacity including:

1. the nature and extent of his property
2. the persons who are natural objects of his bounty,
3. the testamentary provisions he is making, and he must, moreover, be capable of:

   (a) appreciating these factors in relation to each other;
   (b) forming an orderly desire as to the disposition of his property.

Cognitive fluctuations occur in various neurodegenerative disorders but are more commonly noted in delirium and Lewy body dementia [13]. The so-called "lucid interval" and its importance to the capacity assessment is the subject of ongoing legal debate. Some argue that the use of the lucid interval is invalid, arguing that it would be "extremely short in duration, often on the order of seconds or minutes" [13]. As a result, the individual who is being evaluated would not have the sufficient amount of time to appreciate all the relevant factors. If one is experiencing a "lucid interval," it is still within the context of a medical pathophysiological influence that may significantly alter judgment. In cases where an individual has previously made a financial decision (e.g., a will) while in a state of delirium, he may later argue that he had diminished capacity at the time of the financial decision, and that the decision was made when he did not have purpose or knowledge. In post-mortem cases, family members or individuals who would otherwise benefit from the will may similarly contest that will if they are able to provide sufficient evidence to support their case.

Neuroanatomy and Imaging

Rosenbloom et al. [14] clearly outlined how decision-making is dependent on three brain regions:

1. The anterior cingulate cortex (ACC), which organizes conflicting options
2. The dorsolateral prefrontal cortex, which integrates multiple sources of information
3. The orbitofrontal cortex (OFC) and limbic pathways, which are associated with affective-based decisions and reward

It is believed that the more complex the decision-making, the more important the connections between the abovementioned brain regions.

In 2017, Spreng et al. [15] used magnetic resonance imaging (MRI) to compare financially exploited older adults with older adults who were exposed to exploitive situations but were able to identify and avoid it. They found anatomical changes in the financially exploited group, particularly in the anterior insula and posterior superior temporal cortices. These brain regions were noted to have significant roles in affectively based decision-making and social cognition [15–17]. There is also literature describing the impact of decreased insula activity in older adults. They are more likely to rate untrustworthy faces incorrectly [16], increasing the risk for being financial exploited. The OFC and ACC, two of the three main frontal regions in decision-making, have bidirectional connections with the insular and temporal cortices [14]. Individuals with an insular lesion tend to be "indifferent with regard to risky options" [18] or have "emotional bluntness towards risk" [14, 18]. This may resemble apathy, a symptom of MCI and dementia, which may negatively influence the effected individual's ability to correctly assess consequences of decisions [8], including finances.

Relevant Assessment Methods

Grisso and Applebaum have provided legally relevant criteria for decision-making capacity [6]. These can be helpful in assessing financial decision-making capacity. These criteria in making treatment decisions are by far the most commonly used in the assessment of capacity.

1. The individual should clearly indicate the preferred treatment option, where frequent reversals of choice due to a psychiatric or neurologic condition may indicate lack of capacity.
2. The individual should understand relevant information, and this should be demonstrated by the person whose capacity is being questioned.
3. He or she should have the ability to appreciate the situation and its consequences.
4. The person should be able to engage in a rational process of manipulating the relevant information.

Some may argue that an individual who is able to possess the four abilities mentioned above may appropriately have financial capacity and/or testamentary capacity. While not explicitly mentioned in the four elements, evaluators may recognize the individual's vulnerability to undue influence by assessing how well he or she manipulates the relevant information. Nonetheless, the way a lonely, old age individual performs in a structured, formal setting may be different than at home. Therefore, one can demonstrate financial decision-making capacity but still be overwhelmingly vulnerable to financial exploitation.

The Financial Capacity Instrument (FCI) evaluates 9 domains and 18 financial ability tasks, and provides 2 total scores [19]. The FCI has been found to be a reliable assessment tool [20] but contains over 100 items and may take more than an hour to administer [21]. The FCI-Short Form (FCI-SF) measures 37 items and in a concise manner evaluates a range of financial skills in less than 15 minutes [21]. Swanson et al. found that the FCI-SF is sensitive in distinguishing mild cognitive impairment (MCI) and mild Alzheimer's disease dementia [22].

The Lichtenberg Financial Decision Screening Scale (LFDSS) assesses financial decision-making capacity while preventing financial exploitation [23]. The LFDSS consists of ten items, seven of which rate financial decision-making, and three that assess for susceptibility to undue influence. At present, significant limitations of the LFDSS include that it was only studied in a single population group without randomization or blinding.

Lawton and Brody [24, 25] described three levels where an individual of older age may function in regards to financial ability:

1. Level 1 (Independent) — The individual is able to manage his or her finances independently (e.g., can write checks, pays rent, goes to the bank, and is able to budget appropriately).
2. Level 2 (Partially dependent) — Needs help with banking and major purchases but can manage basic day-to-day purchases.
3. Level 3 (Dependent) — The person is not able to handle finances and requires the assistance of others for every financial-related task.

These three levels for financial functioning have not been correlated with vulnerability to financial exploitation (e.g., being particularly vulnerable predatorial fraud and scams). One may hypothetically appear to be independent in financial functioning but may be abnormally incapable of thwarting undue influence.

The Schematic of the Semi-Structured Clinical Interview for Financial Capacity (SCIFC) is a method developed by Marson et al. [26] that guides providers in assessing overall financial capacity and the following eight relevant domains:

1. Basic monetary skills
2. Financial conceptual knowledge
3. Cash transactions
4. Checkbook management
5. Bank statement management
6. Financial judgment
7. Bill payment
8. Knowledge of personal assets and estate arrangements

Even though this interview focuses on domains that can be helpful to understand the financial functioning of an individual, poor performance does not mean that an individual lacks capacity. For instance, if an individual struggled with arithmetic throughout his life and has adequately compensated using a calculator or an accountant, then this could be considered his baseline. Niccolai et al. used the FCI to evaluate 49 persons with MCI and found that semantic arithmetic knowledge is an important cognitive predictor of whether an individual with MCI may lose financial capacity [27]. Nonetheless, the individual whose financial capacity is being called into question may still be able to perform well on Grisso and Applebaum's elements despite poor performance on the SCIFC or FCI.

Widera et al. proposed certain questions that can be included in an informal assessment to probe for potential financial impairment or vulnerability [28]:

General Questions: "Who manages your money, property (and/or investments)?"

"Do you have anyone besides yourself on your checking and savings account?"

"How long has it been like this?"

"Are you having any problems?"

Specific Questions: "Are you having any new problems making change (and/or calculating tips)? "

"When was the last time you were late paying a bill?"

"When was the last time you bounced a check?"

"Have you received any letters or phone calls from your bank with concerns about your account?"

"Has anyone stolen or cheated you out of money?"

Discussion

Accurate assessment of financial capacity is still an area of uncharted territory. It can be challenging to determine an individual's ability to thwart undue influence. Evaluators should be assessing whether the individual has had a significant change in financial management over a specific period of time. For example, the individual who has never donated to a for-profit organization has suddenly started to send them an alarming amount of money, possibly indicating a neurological and/or psychiatric basis for this new behavior. While an individual who has provided donations to a specific charity throughout his or her adult life and has maintained this pattern of giving into late life would not cause the same level of concern.

Family members who are likely to financially benefit from the older individual may be biased and overestimate the individual's financial capacity. Likewise, some family members who raise the issue of impaired financial capacity in their relative may be seeking monetary benefit. An exploitative "friend" or family member may seek the status of payee over an older age individual where funds are spent on the "friend" or family member rather than on the older individual. Some may call the payee in such a circumstance as "a license to exploit." Even though the payee should be discussing the way the money is being spent with the older aged individual, the older individual may overestimate the trustworthiness of the payee and/or have impaired awareness of who is managing his or her finances due to cognitive deficits (e.g., poor memory).

Normal aging (without cognitive impairment) has been associated with an individual's diminished ability to register untrustworthy faces, and therefore increases one's risk for financial exploitation. It is important for the evaluator to keep in mind that certain medications (e.g., anticholinergics, benzodiazepines), polypharmacy, and the use of illicit substances may alter an individual's ability to make rational decisions, including those related to finances. Additionally, in cases where the individual may be accompanied by another individual (e.g., family or friend), the evaluator should ask for that person to step out of the room during the assessment to diminish potential influence. Although collateral information is vital during a financial capacity evaluation, it should not be obtained while assessing the individual whose capacity is being evaluated. The examiner should consider conducting an evaluation over multiple sessions to ensure that the person is providing consistent information.

Older individuals are not likely to be as savvy as the younger generation with using new technology and the internet. As a result, even when an older individual is without cognitive deficits, they may be at increased risk for exploitation through the internet. While the same individual can make appropriate financial decisions, they often are not able to detect an online scam (e.g., a fake bank page that requires your log in information, which then takes all of your funds). One may argue that such a circumstance of financial exploitation is not always an indicator of cognitive impairment. Ethically, providers should balance the concepts of beneficence, where protection is the goal, versus the appreciation of the individual's autonomy [29]. The evaluator's counter-transference and biases may have the potential of influencing the financial capacity assessment by not being able to adequately balance these two ethical concepts. However, it is important to note that there is literature [30] indicating that providers frequently overestimate patients' capacity to make decisions. This overestimation of decision-making capacity in older individuals may lead to detrimental clinical and legal consequences. This overestimation of capacity may be partly due to inadequate training in performing capacity evaluations but also due to administrative or system-based influences.

If an individual is found to lack financial capacity, the court may appoint a guardian or conservator depending on the circumstance and specific state law. Even if an older age individual may appear to have capacity to manage their finances, certain factors such as normal aging, mild cognitive impairment, and loneliness may cause the individual to struggle with dealing of undue influences over their finances. The authors of this chapter are not aware of any validated evaluation tools that focus on an individual's ability to resist undue influence in the setting of making financial decisions. While some individuals may appear to be cognitively intact, they may have impairments in their overall functioning. As a result, it is recommended that evaluators of financial capacity weigh the individual's cognition, emotional state, impulsivity level, and ability to resist undue influence.

Conflicts of Interest or Disclosures   The authors of this book chapter have nothing to disclose and have no conflicts of interest to report.

References

1. Kennedy KM. Testamentary capacity: a practical guide to assessment of ability to make a valid will. J Forensic Leg Med. 2012;19(4):191–5.

2. Caboral-Stevens M, Medetsky M. The construct of financial capacity in older adults. J Gerontol Nurs. 2014;40(8):30–7.
3. Jackson S, Hafemeister T. APS investigation across four types of elder maltreatment. J Adult Prot. 2012;14(2):82–92.
4. Vogel A, Stokholm J, Gade A, Andersen BB, Hejl AM, Waldemar G. Awareness of deficits in mild cognitive impairment and Alzheimer's disease: do MCI patients have impaired insight? Dement Geriatr Cogn Disord. 2004;17(3):181–7.
5. Zamboni G, Drazich E, McCulloch E, Filippini N, Mackay CE, Jenkinson M, et al. Neuroanatomy of impaired self-awareness in Alzheimer's disease and mild cognitive impairment. Cortex. 2013;49(3):668–78.
6. Appelbaum PS. Clinical practice. Assessment of patients' competence to consent to treatment. N Engl J Med. 2007;357(18):1834–40.
7. Vloeberghs R, Opmeer EM, De Deyn PP, Engelborghs S, De Roeck EE. Apathy, depression and cognitive functioning in patients with MCI and dementia. Tijdschr Gerontol Geriatr. 2018;49(3):95–102.
8. Bayard S, Jacus JP, Raffard S, Gely-Nargeot MC. Apathy and emotion-based decision-making in amnesic mild cognitive impairment and Alzheimer's disease. Behav Neurol. 2014;2014:231469.
9. de Mendonca A, Ribeiro F, Guerreiro M, Garcia C. Frontotemporal mild cognitive impairment. J Alzheimers Dis. 2004;6(1):1–9.
10. Stoeckel LE, Stewart CC, Griffith HR, Triebel K, Okonkwo OC, den Hollander JA, et al. MRI volume of the medial frontal cortex predicts financial capacity in patients with mild Alzheimer's disease. Brain Imaging Behav. 2013;7(3):282–92.
11. Yuan P, Raz N. Prefrontal cortex and executive functions in healthy adults: a meta-analysis of structural neuroimaging studies. Neurosci Biobehav Rev. 2014;42:180–92.
12. Tracy VL, Basso MR, Marson DC, Combs DR, Whiteside DM. Capacity for financial decision making in multiple sclerosis. J Clin Exp Neuropsychol. 2017;39(1):46–57.
13. Shulman KI, Hull IM, DeKoven S, Amodeo S, Mainland BJ, Herrmann N. Cognitive fluctuations and the lucid interval in dementia: implications for testamentary capacity. J Am Acad Psychiatry Law. 2015;43(3):287–92.
14. Rosenbloom MH, Schmahmann JD, Price BH. The functional neuroanatomy of decision-making. J Neuropsychiatry Clin Neurosci. 2012;24(3):266–77.

15. Spreng RN, Cassidy BN, Darboh BS, DuPre E, Lockrow AW, Setton R, et al. Financial exploitation is associated with structural and functional brain differences in healthy older adults. J Gerontol A Biol Sci Med Sci. 2017;72(10):1365–8.
16. Samanez-Larkin GR, Knutson B. Decision making in the ageing brain: changes in affective and motivational circuits. Nat Rev Neurosci. 2015;16(5):278–89.
17. Andrews-Hanna JR, Smallwood J, Spreng RN. The default network and self-generated thought: component processes, dynamic control, and clinical relevance. Ann N Y Acad Sci. 2014;1316:29–52.
18. Weller JA, Levin IP, Shiv B, Bechara A. The effects of insula damage on decision-making for risky gains and losses. Soc Neurosci. 2009;4(4):347–58.
19. Griffith HR, Belue K, Sicola A, Krzywanski S, Zamrini E, Harrell L, et al. Impaired financial abilities in mild cognitive impairment: a direct assessment approach. Neurology. 2003;60(3):449–57.
20. Marson DC, Sawrie SM, Snyder S, McInturff B, Stalvey T, Boothe A, et al. Assessing financial capacity in patients with Alzheimer disease: a conceptual model and prototype instrument. Arch Neurol. 2000;57(6):877–84.
21. Gerstenecker A, Eakin A, Triebel K, Martin R, Swenson-Dravis D, Petersen RC, et al. Age and education corrected older adult normative data for a short form version of the Financial Capacity Instrument. Psychol Assess. 2016;28(6):737–49.
22. Swanson C, Marson D, McPherson T, Gerstenecker A, Logovinsky V. The financial capacity instrument - short form is a novel, performance-based measure that may help differentiate mild cognitive impairment and mild dementia due to Alzheimer's disease populations in clinical trials. Alzheimers Dement. 2017;13(7):264–5.
23. Lichtenberg PAPA, Ficker LP, Rahman-Filipiak AM, Tatro RB, Farrell CM, Speir JJM, et al. The Lichtenberg Financial Decision Screening Scale (LFDSS): a new tool for assessing financial decision making and preventing financial exploitation. J Elder Abuse Negl. 2016;28(3):134–51.
24. Marson D. Conceptual models and guidelines for clinical assessment of financial capacity. Arch Clin Neuropsychol. 2016;31(6):541–53.
25. Lawton MP, Brody EM. Assessment of older people: self-maintaining and instrumental activities of daily living. Gerontologist. 1969;9(3):179–86.

26. Marson DC, Martin RC, Wadley V, Griffith HR, Snyder S, Goode PS, et al. Clinical interview assessment of financial capacity in older adults with mild cognitive impairment and Alzheimer's disease. J Am Geriatr Soc. 2009;57(5):806–14.
27. Niccolai LM, Triebel KL, Gerstenecker A, McPherson TO, Cutter GR, Martin RC, et al. Neurocognitive predictors of declining financial capacity in persons with mild cognitive impairment. Clin Gerontol. 2017;40(1):14–23.
28. Widera E, Steenpass V, Marson D, Sudore R. Finances in the older patient with cognitive impairment: "He didn't want me to take over". JAMA. 2011;305(7):698–706.
29. Lichtenberg PA. Financial exploitation, financial capacity, and Alzheimer's disease. Am Psychol. 2016;71(4):312–20.
30. Lepping P. Overestimating patients' capacity. Br J Psychiatry. 2011;199(5):355–6.

Chapter 5
Capacity to Manage Critical Domains of Living: Driving, Voting, and Sexual Expression

Feyza Marouf

Driving

Driving is an essential element of American life that does not diminish with age. Older Americans continue to prefer traveling by private vehicle over any other mode of transport [1]. For most, driving represents independence and vitality, a way to make use of social resources and remain active in their communities [2]. In fact, the elderly are driving more miles per year and keeping their licenses active longer than ever before. By mid-century, roughly a quarter of American drivers will be older adults [3].

Elderly drivers are not more likely to get into accidents than other age groups, but due to their frailty, they are more likely to be fatally injured when a crash occurs [4–6]. To compensate for this risk, many older drivers adopt "self-restricting" driving strategies [7]. They avoid driving in bad weather, heavy traffic or in difficult road conditions. They prefer local

F. Marouf (✉)
Massachusetts General Hospital, Boston, MA, USA

Harvard Medical School, Boston, MA, USA
e-mail: Fmarouf@mgh.harvard.edu

© Springer Nature Switzerland AG 2019
M. Balasubramaniam et al. (eds.), *Psychiatric Ethics in Late-Life Patients*, https://doi.org/10.1007/978-3-030-15172-0_5

trips rather than traveling long distances, and daytime hours rather than driving at night [8]. Generally, they are more responsible than other age groups; more likely to wear seat belts and less likely to drink and drive [1].

According to TRIP, a national transportation research group, more than 600,000 people aged 70 or older stop driving each year [9]. Women are more likely to cease driving than men of similar age and with the same levels of illness and disability [10]. When driving stops, older adults make fewer visits to friends and family, take fewer trips to the doctor, shopping centers and religious activities [11]. Dependency on others to meet transportation needs can strain relationships. In the midst of such tensions and social isolation, there is an increased risk of depression, anxiety, and nursing home placement [12, 13].

Regulating Safety

Many states attempt to identify, assess and regulate older drivers by requiring them to renew their drivers' licenses and pass visual tests at more frequent intervals than younger age groups [14, 15]. Some states prohibit renewal by mail, requiring elderly drivers to appear in person. In other states, drivers are required to take a road test for license renewal or must supply a doctor's approval [16, 17]. In one study, a mandate for in-person license renewal for older adults was associated with a 31% reduction in fatal crash involvement rates for drivers aged 85 and older [18].

The risk of motor vehicle accidents is significantly increased for the cognitively impaired older adults. Drivers with Alzheimer's dementia are up to four times more likely to be involved in motor vehicle collisions when compared to healthy age-matched controls [19, 20]. Driving is also unpredictable and potentially unsafe among older adults with Parkinson's and Lewy Body dementias, who suffer more motor dysfunction, as well as drivers with frontotemporal dementia who may display early executive dysfunction and disinhibition, as well as impulsivity and anger [21–23].

Therefore, guidelines suggest that individuals with moderate to severe dementia should not drive [24–27]. While there is no clear recommendation for persons with mild cognitive impairments, these drivers are more likely than age-matched controls to exhibit impaired driving performance and to fail road tests, although the risk of actual crashes is unknown [28, 29].

Clinician Advice

Despite the available guidelines, many clinicians hesitate to initiate conversations about driving ability with elderly individuals. There can be concerns about restricting the patient autonomy, interfering with the quality of life and disrupting the doctor–patient relationship [30, 31]. As only 2% of older Americans make trips by public transit, loss of driving ability can have a profound impact on their activity levels. This is particularly true for older Americans who live in rural areas, where limited transit options are available [32]. Accordingly, angry and defensive reactions by individuals are common [33].

Clinicians can reduce the conflict by validating the reality of the life disruption caused by driving cessation and focusing on driving skills, rather than the individual's age to frame the discussion of safety [34, 35]. Helping individuals plan for "driving retirement" might involve a social worker or community organization to identify the types of transportation options available, including public transit, ride services, and private arrangements [36]. Ideally, this sort of planning occurs well before the mobility situation becomes urgent.

Capacity Evaluation

Clinicians frequently find themselves in the challenging position of evaluating capacity to drive in elderly individuals [37]. In fact, recommendation by their doctor is the most cited reason for older adults to stop driving [38]. Capacity assessments are usually made in clinic, where clinicians are in a unique position to observe and weigh potential dangers against individual circumstances [39]. The clinician's evaluation may report a range of cognitive and physical functioning, and conclude that someone is safe to drive, that more testing is needed, that driving should be reduced in the near future, or that driving should stop [40]. The state uses this information to make a final legal determination of *yes* or *no* in terms of fitness to drive.

Clinicians assess the capacity to drive by integrating evidence of relevant conditions, risks, abilities, limitations, and potential supports to the driver [41]. Such an evaluation usually begins by taking a careful driving history, including frequency of driving, location, length and reason for trips, types of roadways used, familiarity with roadways, frequency of night driving, rush hour and freeway driving, use of a navigator, presence of caregivers who can drive, caregivers' perceptions of driving skills, types of passengers transported, and record of crashes, tickets, near misses and episodes of getting lost while driving [25, 42].

Additionally, clinicians record medical conditions that can impair driving ability, especially those that have the potential to improve with treatment or accommodations [43, 44]. This can include dementia, delirium, diabetes, stroke, psychiatric disorders, changes in vision due to cataracts, glaucoma, macular degeneration, and diabetic retinopathy, or limitations in movement due to arthritis [45,46]. Medications also frequently impair driving ability. The use of long-acting benzodiazepines is associated with increased crash rates in older adults. Opioids, sedating antidepressants, hypnotics, antipsychotics, antihistamines, glaucoma agents, NSAIDs and muscle relaxants also contribute to increasing difficulty with driving [47].

Notably, cognitive tests like the Mini-Mental State Examination (MMSE) and the Montreal Cognitive Assessment (MOCA) are not predictive of driving risk or motor vehicle crashes and cannot be used to identify unsafe drivers [48, 49]. In the absence of standardized tests, clinicians frequently refer individuals with mild cognitive impairment to a driving specialist, usually an occupational therapist based in a hospital or a rehabilitation center. These evaluations are off-road tests that can be expensive [50]. When there is high suspicion of impaired capacity, including concern for moderate to severe dementia, the clinical recommendation is usually for a performance-based road test at the local motor vehicles department [51].

Legal Obligations

Clinicians reporting of impaired drivers have been shown to reduce the risk of collisions [38]. Given the state to state differences between optional and required reporting requirements, obtaining a consultation with an attorney or the local risk management department is usually advised before filing an official report. Although physicians may face personal liability for their reports, most states provide physicians with specific legal protections for doing so. Some states also prohibit the department of motor vehicles from disclosing the name of the reporting physician to the patient [52].

When a clinician submits a report, the department of motor vehicles contacts the older driver to schedule a fitness to drive evaluation, usually a performance-based road test. These tests focus on particular difficulties that elderly drivers face, including driving too slowly, failing to recognize traffic signs, driving off the road and not braking properly. Road tests assess for ability to check and change lanes, merging, turning left, signal to park, and follow a route. However, such evaluations are rarely standardized, and the data supporting their use are limited [53].

In a study by Duchek, 88% of drivers with very mild dementia and 69% of drivers with mild dementia were still able to pass a formal road test [29]. Yet, very few (less than 4%) of older adults referred to driving evaluations by physicians will retain their driver's licenses [54]. The referrals themselves may represent the first step of a de-licensing process. In this context, it is not surprising that many older drivers regret and resist the recommendation to stop driving once it made. In fact, roughly a third of cognitively impaired drivers continue to drive [55]. Even license suspension does not necessarily stop these elders from driving, reflecting the remarkable importance of driving even among the cognitively impaired.

Voting

The act of voting is an inalienable right employed frequently in late life. Older voters feel empowered and involved when participating in elections [56]. They tend to vote in larger proportions than any other age group. In the 2016 presidential election, for example, the turnout for citizens aged 65–74 was 70.9% [57]. This level of political participation allows elderly voters to play a pivotal role in election results. Consider that the outcome of the 2000 American presidential election was decided by just 537 votes in Florida, the state with the highest percentage of seniors.

Older adults tend to view voting as a responsibility. They vote on a range of issues, not only topics associated with aging [58]. Despite this degree of civic engagement, many older adults are limited from voting by their health status [59]. Voting is a multistep process, involving both physical and cognitive functioning. Voters must update their registration information, request forms, meet deadlines, and travel to a polling place. Voting often requires a form of photo identification, which 18% of voters older than 65 do not possess [60].

Elderly persons who maintain their cognitive functioning are more likely to vote than those who experience cognitive decline [61]. A recent Finnish study revealed that among a range of major diseases, dementia had the strongest negative correlation with voting [62]. Yet, the cognitively impaired elderly continue to vote, especially in the earliest stages of dementia. A survey of 100 individuals diagnosed with dementia who attended a memory clinic found that 60% had voted in a recent American election. The vast majority did so in a polling booth by themselves [63].

Gatekeepers

The role of the caregiver is quite important with regard to voting. Spousal caregivers may raise the likelihood of a care recipient voting, especially if the caregiver agrees that even cognitively impaired individuals should be allowed to vote [64]. However, older adults with dementia who remain capable of voting may be prevented from doing so by caregivers who incorrectly assume that they lack capacity. Caregivers may also decide not to inform an elderly person of the right to vote, refuse to supply a registration form or fail to assist the person in voting [65].

Compromising the integrity of elections, caregivers sometimes cast ballots on behalf of demented individuals, whether from beneficent or dishonorable motives, without their knowledge or against their wishes [66]. Terms such as "patient" or "nursing home resident" imply dependence on the caregiver and can embolden the caregiver's sense of paternalism. This is in contrast to referring to elderly voters, even those with cognitive decline, as "taxpaying consumers" [67].

Studies of nursing homes reveal that staff frequently screen residents themselves to determine who has the capacity to vote before allowing elderly residents to vote or assisting them to vote [68]. Few state guidelines exist for voting in long-term care facilities with regard to promoting participation and limiting fraud. Notably, the completion of absentee ballots in nursing homes is not regulated and varies widely across different facilities, despite the prevalence of absentee voting among elderly voters [69].

Many states allow political operatives to distribute absentee voter applications to residents in nursing homes, as well as assist in completing and collecting ballots without requiring a witness to be legally present [70]. A study comparing voting practices in several Maryland counties suggests that directly involving election officials with long term care staff improves voter registration and voter turnout. In nursing home settings, assigning responsibility to election officials to notify staff of relevant deadlines, as well to deliver ballots and supervise polling booths could reduce the opportunities for fraud [71, 72].

Voting Facilitation

In recent decades, Congress has made efforts to promote accessibility for voters with disabilities, most notably through the Voting Accessibility for the Elderly and Handicapped Act of 1984, the Americans with Disabilities Act of 1990, and the Help America Vote Act of 2002. The American Bar Association has urged federal, state, local governments "to improve the administration of elections to facilitate voting by all individuals with disabilities, including people with cognitive impairments." Recognizing the demographic shifts ahead, the American Election Administration Commission noted in 2015 that roughly a third of voters will need some form of voting assistance by 2050.

Voting assistance includes help with transportation to voting sites, access into buildings, wheelchair accommodations, visual needs, and clear, simplified instructions on how to vote. Few of the current electronic or optical scanning systems are tailored to people with cognitive impairment [73]. More effective ballot design may reduce confusion in the polling booth, including providing pictures of the candidates. The capability of older adults with cognitive impairment to learn new techniques, including the most popular electronic voting machines, is not well understood. Many elderly voters retain the ability to vote using older skills, such as pulling a lever or punching a card [73].

States vary widely in their implementation of voting facilitation, including absentee voting, early voting, voter identification and same day registration [74]. Early voting can be especially helpful in providing flexibility to elderly voters, but can complicate the costs of running a local election. Mobile voting allows bipartisan pairs of election officials to bring ballots directly to long-term care facilities, where they can assist voters and register new voters. Mobile voting is allowed in 23 states, but laws vary on whether state or local officials are responsible for administering this system [75].

In a survey conducted over 11 years across 30 European countries, Wass et al. found that among voters with health problems or activity limitations, the higher the level of voting facilitation, the lower the turnout [76]. In fact, voting facilitation had almost no effect on the voting patterns of healthy adults. Instead, there was a negative influence on individuals with poor health or limited ability. In Wass's study, only proxy voting relatively increased participation among those with activity limitations. In the United States, however, proxy voting is not legally permitted.

Capacity Evaluation

Unlike driving, voting has not been identified as a public health problem. Quite to the contrary— participation in elections increases self-esteem and a sense of independence, reinforcing democratic principles and enabling even vulnerable groups to challenge imbalances of power [56]. No state requires that a physician notify the state's voting board about a patient who lacks the capacity to vote. In addition, there is no easily administered, validated test to determine voting ability. In fact, many people with cognitive decline retain their capacity to vote [77].

State laws vary substantially in their approach to voting capacity assessment. In some states, older adults with dementia are not allowed to vote until legally deemed to have the capacity to vote. Yet other states do not have any voting competency standards [78]. Many states have adopted the recommendation of the American Bar Association: "If you can communicate, with or without accommodations, a choice to vote, you are competent to vote." However, not all persons who want to vote understand the nature and effect of voting [79].

A desire to vote has been found to be a poor predictor of voting capacity. Whereas most individuals with mild dementia retain the capacity to vote, those with more severe illness do not. The severity of dementia generally correlates with the decreasing capacity to vote. Moderate dementia is most variable in terms of voting abilities and frequently the hardest to assess [80]. The use of a structured tool such as the Competence

Assessment Tool for Voting (CAT-V) that focuses on four standard decision-making abilities: understanding, appreciation, reasoning and making a choice, improves the assessment of an individual's capacity to vote.

Older adults who are deemed mentally incompetent, incapacitated or under guardianship are frequently disenfranchised from voting despite the fact that they may be well informed about election issues even if they need help with other areas of functioning [78]. In Doe vs. Rowe, a federal district court in Maine ruled that a person under guardianship retains the capacity to vote if he or she understands the nature and effect of voting and is able to choose among candidates and questions on the ballot [81]. This ruling does not hold the voter to a higher standard than other populations. Rather, under this ruling older adults retain the right to vote unless explicitly prohibited by the terms of their guardianship.

Sexual Expression

The sexual needs of older adults are frequently minimized in our culture. Older adults are less likely to discuss their sexual activity with their clinicians than younger individuals. Providers often take a limited sexual history due to their own misconceptions [82, 83]. In nursing homes, expectations can be that of abstinence. Yet, basic needs for pleasure and connection do not diminish with age. Rather, sexuality remains an important measure of quality of life across the lifespan [84, 85].

Studies show that sexual activity in older adults can increase self-esteem, boost cognitive functioning, improve relationships, and cultivate independence [86]. Sexual instincts also survive cognitive decline. Among the cognitively impaired, for whom verbal expression can be difficult, touch and intimacy are important ways to maintain communication, provide a sense of emotional well-being, offer relief from stress, and cultivate feelings of warmth and safety [87].

Cognitive Decline and Sexuality

During the initial stages of dementia, sexual expression may increase due to disinhibition or decrease as a form of apathy. Sexually inappropriate behaviors occur in all stages of dementia, as well as with mild cognitive impairment. The emergence of inappropriate sexual behaviors often complicates the course of dementia [88, 89]. Early in the course of illness, individuals with Parkinson's dementia may show poor impulse control while those with Frontotemporal dementia can exhibit hypersexuality [90, 91].

Evaluation of these behaviors includes diagnostic clarification to rule out delirium or underlying medical etiology, careful assessment of any mood disorder, delusions, substance use, attention-seeking behavior or long-standing personality traits. The management of inappropriate sexual behaviors usually starts with non-pharmacological strategies, including removal of precipitants, distraction strategies, and offering other opportunities to relieve sexual urges [92]. Discontinuing medications that worsen disinhibition is also important. While antidepressants can be useful in reducing libido, the side effects of antipsychotics usually outweigh the benefits, and the use of hormonal treatments is controversial [93].

Moral Dilemmas

Partners of those living with dementia face numerous challenges. Frequently, spouses are primary caregivers attempting to balance the changing needs of their impaired partners with their own desires [94, 95]. Moral dilemmas become numerous, as exemplified by the 2015 case of Henry Rayhons, a former state legislator who faced a felony charge for accusations of sexual abuse toward his wife, an individual with Alzheimer's disease, after staff members decided she was too cognitively impaired to consent to sex. Mr. Rayhons was found not guilty in a jury trial, but the case ignited debate about whether staff, doctors, or even adult children acting as guardians, have better ability to judge the enjoyment of a demented patient than the spouse in questions [96, 97].

Protecting cognitively impaired individuals from unwanted, distressing, or exploitative sexual encounters is critical. Rates of abuse may be higher for older adults living in nursing homes versus those in the community. Only 1 in 24 cases of elder abuse is reported according to the World Health Organization [98]. Signs of abuse can include weight loss, bruises, broken bones, and increased confusion. However, evaluation of these signs in older adults with dementia can be difficult. In addition, in one study, elderly victims displayed fear or ambivalence toward the abuser in only half of cases and were less likely when compared to other age groups to report instances of abuse [99].

Capacity Evaluation

There is no medical standard for evaluation of the ability to consent to sex in late life. Requests for capacity assessments are made in cases of sexual assault, including both criminal charges against individuals and the civil liability of nursing homes for their residents. Courts usually consider awareness, understanding, and voluntariness as the three main determinants of capacity to consent to sexual activity [100]. Ethical principles focus on finding a balance between autonomy, beneficence, non-maleficence, and safety. Some states require not just an understanding of sex, but also the moral and social implications of sexual behaviors, including impact on other relationships [101].

The demented elderly are particularly vulnerable to losing the capacity to consent to sex [102]. The presence of delusions or misidentification complicates the determination of awareness. Tarzia et al. have suggested that interfering in a sexual relationship between people who are otherwise content is recommended only if the participants are not aware of the true identity of their partners, believing that person to be someone else; for instance, their spouse [103]. In order to have capacity for sex, the risks of sexual activity also need to be understood. This includes varied risks as falling out of bed, contracting sexually transmitted disease, and struggling with a sense of abandonment when the relationship ends [104].

In a 2013 survey of over 300 nursing home directors, the Society for Post-Acute and Long Term Care Medicine found that more than two-thirds identified sexual concerns in their facilities, roughly half noted sexual activity between residents, but the majority had no specific policies in place about sexual behaviors [105, 106]. Study of intervention by ombudsmen in long-term care highlights the need for resident advocates to support residents' rights. Standards of practice should include decision-making procedures for ethically complex situations, occurrences of sexual abuse, and inappropriate sexual activity [107, 108].

The Hebrew Home in Riverdale, NY, is an example of a facility with specific guidelines for assessing sexual consent capacity, including interdisciplinary team assessment of verbal and non-verbal communications of pleasure, mood before and after sexual contact, and understanding of the personal meaning of sexual activity, including previous patterns of sexual behavior [109]. The goals of these policies are to uphold autonomy and sexual rights while also protecting residents under both state and federal law. Both best interest and substituted judgment standards are utilized for someone deemed incapable of providing sexual consent [110].

Conclusions

Capacity assessments in late life can involve very personal aspects of living, including choosing a sexual partner, voting for a candidate in election, or driving a private car at night. Evaluating the capacity to engage in these activities requires a clinician to act in a person's best interest (beneficience) and avoid harm (maleficence). Clinicians must integrate complex clinical data, including medical conditions, cognitive abilities, functional skills, personal values, and past behaviors with an analysis of the risks at hand and an understanding of the legal standards. This formulation must be weighed against the ethical principle of self-determination (autonomy), which includes the right to make bad decisions.

Difficult capacity assessments often involve individuals who fall into moderate ranges of cognitive impairment. The lack of specific guidelines for clinicians in this "gray area" can make evaluations quite complicated, especially given the expectation that clinicians conclude with a "yes or no" answer regarding capacity. To offer the most careful assessment, clinicians should be aware of their own biases, including comfort tolerating risk. By being informed about potential accommodations and types of community services available, considering harm reduction models and cultural influences, clinicians can help initiate conversations, identify patient and family preferences, and make plans in advance of cognitive, mental or physical decline, without over-emphasizing the authority to direct care (paternalism).

Many individuals with diminished capacity are currently managed by family members or caregivers without any formal capacity assessment. Judicial review occurs rarely for driving capacity, very rarely for sexual consent capacity (usually only with litigation), and extremely rarely in the case of voting capacity (in most states voting rights are retained even under guardianship) [111]. As baby boomers age and cognitive impairment becomes increasingly prevalent in society, it is likely that formal requests for capacity evaluations will increase in an effort to maintain safety on the roads, mobilize voters during elections, and ensure against sexual abuse in nursing homes. There is a strong need for more research to help guide this expanding and difficult area of clinical practice.

References

1. Retchin SM, Anapolle J. An overview of the older driver. Clin Geriatr Med. 1993;9:279–96.
2. Delling AM, Segal M, Sleet DM, Barrett-Connor E. Driving cessation: what older former drivers tell us. J Am Geriatr Soc. 2001;49:431–5.

3. Foley DJ, Heimovitz HK, Guralnik JA, Brock DB. Driving life expectancy of persons aged 70 years and older in the United States. Am J Public Health. 2002;92:1284–9.
4. Wang CC, Carr DB. Older driver safety: a report from the older drivers project. J Am Geriatr Soc. 2004;52:143–9.
5. Rollison JJ, Hewson PJ, Hellier E, et al. Risk of fatal injury in older adult drivers, passengers, and pedestrians. J Am Geriatr Soc. 2012;60(8):1504–8.
6. Cicchino JB, McCartt AT. Trends in older driver crash involvement rates and survivability in the United States: an update. Accid Anal Prev. 2014;72:44–54.
7. Ragland DR, Satariano WA, MacLeod KE. Reasons given by older people for limitation or avoidance of driving. Gerontologist. 2004;44:237–44.
8. Baldock MR, Mathias JL, McLean J, Berndt A. Self-regulation and driving and older drivers' abilities. Clin Gerontol. 2006;30:53–66.
9. 2018 TRIP report: preserving the mobility and safety of older Americans. www.tripnet.org/docs/Older_Americans_Mobility_Trip_Report_2018.pdf. Accessed 10 Dec 2018.
10. Kostyniuk LP, Molnar LJ. Self-regulatory driving practices among older adults: health, age and sex effects. Accid Anal Prev. 2008;4(4):1576–80.
11. Marottoli RA, Glass TA, Williams CS, Cooney LM Jr, Berkman LF, de Leon CFM. Consequences of driving cessation: decreased out-of-home activity levels. J Gerontol B Psychol Sci Soc Sci. 2000;55(6):S334–40.
12. Fonda SJ, Wallace RB, Herzog AR. Changes in driving patterns and worsening depressive symptoms among older adults. J Gerontol B Psychol Sci Soc Sci. 2001;56(6):S343–51.
13. Freeman EE, Gange SJ, Murioz B, West SK. Driving status and risk of entry into long-term care in older adults. Am J Public Health. 2006;96(7):1254–9.
14. Grabowski DC, Campbell CM, Morrisey MA. Elderly licensure laws and motor vehicle fatalities. JAMA. 2004; 291(23):2840–6.
15. Langford J, Bohensky M, Koppel S, Newstead S. Do age-based mandatory assessments reduce older drivers' risk to other road users? Accid Anal Prev. 2008;40(6):1913–8.
16. Levy DT, Vernick JS, Howard KA. Relationship between driver's license renewal policies and fatal crashes involving drivers 70 years or older. JAMA. 1995;274(13):1026–30.

17. Dugan E, Barton KN, Coyle C, Lee CM. U.S. policies to enhance older driver safety: a systematic review of the literature. J Aging Soc Policy. 2013;25:335–52.

18. Tefft BC. Driver license renewal policies and fatal crash involvement rates of older drivers, United States, 1986–2011. Inj Epidemiol. 2014;1(1):25.

19. Carr DB, O'Neill D. Mobility and safety issues in drivers with dementia. Int Psychogeriatr. 2015;27(10):1613–22.

20. Chee JN, Rapoport MJ, Molnar F, Herrmann N, O'Neill D, Marottoli R, et al. Update on the risk of motor vehicle collision or driving impairment with dementia: a collaborative international systematic review and meta-analysis. Am J Geriatr Psychiatry. 2017;25(12):1376–90.

21. Emre M, Ford PJ, Bilgic B, Uc EY. Cognitive impairment and dementia in Parkinson's disease: practical issues and management. Mov Disord. 2014;29(5):663–72.

22. Yasmin S, Stinchcombe A, Gagnon S. Driving competence in mild dementia with Lewy bodies: in search of cognitive predictors using driving simulation. Int J Alzheimers Dis. 2015;2015:806024.

23. Turk K, Dugan E. Research brief: a literature review of frontotemporal dementia and driving. Am J Alzheimers Dis Other Demen. 2014;29(5):404–8.

24. Reger MA, Welsh RK, Watson GS, et al. The relationship between neuropsychological functioning and driving ability in dementia: a meta-analysis. Neuropsychology. 2004; 18:85–93.

25. Carr DB, Ott BR. The older adult driver with cognitive impairment. JAMA. 2010;303(16):1632–41.

26. Rapoport MJ, Chee JN, Carr DB, et al. An international approach to enhancing a national guideline on driving and dementia. Curr Psychiatry Rep. 2018;20(16):16–25.

27. Iverson DJ, Gronseth GS, Reger MA, Classen S, Dubinsky RM, Rizzo M. Practice parameter update: evaluation and management of driving risk in dementia: report of the quality standards Subcommittee of the American Academy of Neurology. Neurology. 2010;74(16):1316–24.

28. Vaughan L, Hogan PE, Rapp SR, Dugan E, Marottoli RA, Snively BM, et al. Driving with mild cognitive impairment or dementia: cognitive test performance and proxy report of daily life function in older women. J Am Geriatr Soc. 2015;63(9):1774–82.

29. Duchek JM, Carr DB, Hunt L, et al. Longitudinal driving performance in early stage dementia of the Alzheimer type. J Am Geriatr Soc. 2003;51(10):1342–7.
30. Persson D. The elderly driver: deciding when to stop. The Gerontologist. 1993;33(1):88–91.
31. Betz ME, Jones J, Carr DB. System facilitators and barriers to discussing older driver safety in primary care settings. Inj Prev. 2014;21(4):231–7.
32. Dye CJ, Willoughby DF, Battisto DG. Advice from rural elders: what it takes to age in place. Educ Gerontol. 2011;37(1):74–93.
33. Byszewski AM, Molnar FJ, Aminzadeh F. The impact of disclosure of unfitness to drive in persons with newly diagnosed dementia: patient and caregiver perspectives. Clin Gerontol. 2010;33(2):152–63.
34. D'Ambrosio LA, Coughlin JF, Mohyde M, Carruth A, Hunter JC, Stern RA. Caregiver communications and the transition from driver to passenger among people with dementia. Top Geriatr Rehabil. 2009;25(1):33–42.
35. Jenkins D, Holston EC. Conceptualizing the choice of driving retirement by older adults. Top Geriatr Rehabil. 2015;1(2):90–7.
36. Liddle J, Bennett S, Allen S, Lie DC, Standen B, Pachana NA. The stages of driving cessation for people with dementia: needs and challenges. Int Psychogeriatr. 2013;25:2033–46.
37. Reuben DB, Silliman RA, Traines M. The aging driver, medicine, policy, and ethics. J Am Geriatr Soc. 1988;36:1135–42.
38. Redelmeier DA, Yarnell CJ, Thiruchelvam D, Tibshirani RJ. Physicians' warnings for unfit drivers and the risk of trauma from road crashes. N Engl J Med. 2012;367(13):1228–36.
39. Jang RW, Man-Son-Hing M, Molnar FJ, et al. Family physicians' attitudes and practice regarding assessments of medical fitness to drive in older persons. J Gen Intern Med. 2007;22:531–43.
40. Molnar FJ, Rapoport MJ, Roy M. Driving and dementia: maximizing the utility of in-office screening and assessment tools. Can Geriatr Soc J CME. 2012;2(2):11–4.
41. Carmody J, Traynor V, Iverson D. Dementia and driving: an approach for general practice. Aust Fam Physician. 2012;41(4):230–3.
42. Frank CC, Lee L, Molnar F. Driving assessment for people with dementia. Can Fam Physician. 2018;64(10):744.
43. MacLeod KE, Satariano WA, Ragland DR. The impact of health problems on driving status among older adults. J Trans Health. 2014;1(2):86–94.

44. Ball K, Owsley C, Stalvey B, Roenker DL, Sloane ME, Graves M. Driving avoidance and functional impairment in older drivers. Accid Anal Prev. 1998;30:313–22.
45. Campbell MK, Bush TL, Hale WE. Medical conditions associated with driving cessation in community-dwelling, ambulatory elders. J Gerontol. 1993;48(4):S230–4.
46. Gruber N, Mosimann UP, Muri RM, Nef T. Vision and night driving abilities of elder drivers. Traffic Inj Prev. 2013;14:477–85.
47. McGwin G Jr, Sims RV, Pulley L, Roseman JM. Relations among chronic medical conditions, medications, and automobile crashes in the elderly: a population-based case–control study. Am J Epidemiol. 2000;152:424–31.
48. Hollis AM, Duncanson H, Kapust LR, Xi PM, O'Connor MG. Validity of the mini-mental state examination and the Montreal cognitive assessment in the prediction of driving test outcome. J Am Geriatr Soc. 2015;63(5):988–92.
49. Vaughan L, Hogan PE, Rapp SR, Dugan E, Marottoli RA, Snively BM, et al. Driving with mild cognitive impairment or dementia: cognitive test performance and proxy report of daily life function in older women. J Am Geriatr Soc. 2015;63(9):1774–82. Korner-Bitensky N, Bitensky J, Sofer S, Man-Son-Hing M, Gelinas I. Driving evaluation practices of clinicians working in the United States and Canada. Am J Occup Ther. 2006;60(4):428–434.
50. Martin AJ, Marottoli R, O'Neill D. Driving assessment for maintaining mobility and safety in drivers with dementia. Cochrane Database Syst Rev. 2009;(1):CD006222.
51. Molnar FJ, Byszewski AM, Rapoport M, Dalziel WB. Practical experience-based approaches to assessing fitness to drive in dementia. Geriatr Aging. 2009;12(2):83–92.
52. Rapoport MJ, Herrmann N, Molnar FJ, et al. Sharing the responsibility for as sessing the risk of the driver with dementia. CMAJ. 2007;177(6):599–601.
53. Brown LB, Ott BR, Papandonatos GD, Sui Y, Ready RE, Morris JC. Prediction of on-road driving performance in patients with early Alzheimer's disease. J Am Geriatr Soc. 2005;53:94–8.
54. Meuser TM, Carr DB, Ulfarsson GF. Motor-vehicle crash history and licensing outcomes for older drivers reported as medically impaired in Missouri. Accid Anal Prev. 2009;41(2):246–52.
55. Kennedy GJ. Advanced age, dementia, and driving: guidance for the patient, family and physician. Prim Psychiatry. 2009;16(9):19–23.

56. Arah OA. Effect of voting abstention and life course socioeconomic position on self-reported health. J Epidemiol Community Health. 2008;62(8):759–60.

57. United States Census Bureau. https://www.census.gov/newsroom/blogs/random-samplings/2017/05/voting_in_america.html.

58. Goerres A. Why are older people more likely to vote? The impact of aging on electoral turnout in Europe. Br J Politics Int Relat. 2007;9:90–121.

59. Burden BC, et al. How different forms of health matter to political participation. J Polit. 2017;79(1):166–78.

60. Hudson N, McRory B, Regan P. Do your individuals need help to access the ballot box? Nurs Times. 2010;106(15):8.

61. Pérès KC, Helmer H, Amieva JM, et al. Natural history of decline in instrumental activities of daily living performance over the 10 years preceding the clinical diagnosis of dementia: a prospective population-based study. J Am Geriatr Soc. 2008;56(1):37–44.

62. Sund R, Lahtinen H, Wass H, et al. How voter turnout varies between different chronic conditions? A population-based register study. J Epidemiol Community Health. 2017;71:475–9.

63. Ott BR, Heindel WC, Papadonatos GD. A survey of voter participation by cognitively impaired elderly patients. Neurology. 2003;60(9):1546–8.

64. Karlawish JH, Casarett DA, James RD, Propert KJ, Asch DA. Do persons with dementia vote? Neurology. 2002;58:1100–2.

65. Fay JA. Elderly electors go postal: ensuring absentee ballot integrity for older voters. Elder LJ. 2005;13:453–5.

66. Tokaji D, Colker R. Absentee voting by people with disabilities: promoting access and integrity. McGeorge Law Rev. 2007;38:1015–634.

67. Jones P, Dawson P. 'Choice' in collective decision-making processes: instrumental or expressive approval? J Socio-Economics. 2007;36(1):102–17.

68. Karlawish JH, Bonnie RJ, Appelbaum PS, et al. Identifying the barriers and challenges to voting by residents in nursing homes and assisted living settings. J Aging Soc Policy. 2008;20:65–79.

69. Nabi W. Voting practices of residents of nursing and residential homes. J Geriatr Psychiatry. 2002;17(6):589–90.

70. Karlawish JH, Bonnaie RJ, Appelbaum PS, et al. Addressing the ethical, legal and social issues raised by voting by persons with dementia. J Am Med Assoc. 2004;292(11):1345–50.

71. Rosenblatt A, Samus QM, Steele CD, Baker AS, Harper MG, et al. The Maryland Assisted Living Study: prevalence, recognition, and treatment of dementia and other psychiatric disorders in the assisted living population of Central Maryland. J Am Geriatr Soc. 2004;52(10):1618–25.

72. Karlawish J, Appelbaum PS, Bonnie R, Karlan P, McConnell S. Policy statement on voting by persons with dementia residing in long-term care facilities. Alzheimer's Dement. 2006;2:243–5.

73. Sabatino C, Spurgeon E. Facilitating voting as people age: implications of cognitive impairment. McGeorge Law Rev. 2007;38:843–59.

74. Pacheco J, Fletcher J. Incorporating health into studies of political behavior: evidence for turnout and partisanship. Polit Res Q. 2015;68:104–16.

75. Grady D, Karlawish JH, Sabatino C, Markowitz D, et al. Bringing the vote to the residents of long-term care facilities: a study of the benefits and challenges of mobile polling. Election Law J. 2011;10(1):5–14.

76. Wass H, Mattila M, Rapeli L, Soderlund P. Voting while ailing? The effect of voter facilitation instruments on health-related differences in turnout. JEPOP. 2017;27(4):503–22.

77. Karlawish JH, Bonnie RJ. Voting by elderly persons with cognitive impairment: lessons from other democratic nations. McGeorges Law Rev. 2007;38:879–916.

78. Wislowski A, Cuellar N. Voting rights for older Americans with dementia: implications for health care providers. Nurs Outlook. 2006;54(2):68–73.

79. Appelbaum P, Bonnie R, Karlawish JH. The capacity to vote of persons with Alzheimer's dementia. Am J Psychiatry. 2005;162:2094–100.

80. Irastorza LJ, Corujo P, Banuelos P. Capacity to vote in person with dementia and the elderly. Int J Alzheimer's Dis. 2011;11:1–6.

81. Doe v. Rowe. Decision by a Maine Federal District court. 2001. Retrieved from https://www.med.uscourts.gov/opinions/Singal/2001/GZS_08092001_1- 00cv206_DOE_v_ROWE.pdf.

82. Lindau ST, Schumm LP, Laumann EO, Levinson W, Waite LJ. A study of sexuality and health among older adults in the United States. N Engl J Med. 2007;357:762–74.

83. Rheaume C, Mittym E. Sexuality and intimacy in older adults. Geriatr Nurs. 2008;9(5):342–9.

84. Gott M, Hinchliff S. How important is sex in later life? The views of older people. Soc Sci Med. 2003;56:1617–28.
85. Abenbow SM, Beeston D. Sexuality, aging and dementia. Int Psychogeriatr. 2012;24(7):1026–33.
86. Lindau ST, Gavrilova N. Sex, health, and years of sexually active life gained due to good health: evidence from two US population based cross sectional surveys of aging. BMJ. 2010;340:810.
87. Dourado M, Finamore C, Barroso MF, Santos R, Laks J. Sexual satisfaction in dementias: perspectives of patients and spouses. Sex Disabil. 2010;28(3):195–203.
88. Torrisi M, Cacciola A, Marra A, et al. Inappropriate behaviors and hyper sexuality in individuals with dementia: an overview of a neglected issue. Geriatr Gerontol Int. 2017;27:865–74.
89. Tucker IL. Management of inappropriate sexual behaviors in dementia: a literature review. Int Psychogeriatr. 2010;22(5):683–92.
90. Cooper CA, Jadidian A, Paggi M, Romrell J, Okun MS, Rodriguez RL, Fernandez HH, et al. Prevalence of hyper sexual behavior in Parkinson's disease patients: not restricted to males and dopamine agonist use. Int J Gen Med. 2009;2:576–61.
91. Tsatali M, Tsolaki MN, Christodoulou TP, Papaliagkas VT. The complex nature of inappropriate sexual behaviors in patients with dementia: can we put it into a frame? Sex Disabil. 2011;29:143–56.
92. Joller P, Gupta N, Seitz DP, Frank C, Gibson M, Gill SS. Approach to inappropriate sexual behavior in people with dementia. Can Fam Physician. 2013;59:255–60.
93. Kyomen HH, Nobel KW, Wei JY. The use of estrogen to decrease aggressive physical behavior in elderly men with dementia. J Am Geriatr Soc. 1991;57(11):2161–2.
94. Ballard C, Solis M, Gahir M, Cullen P, George S, Oyebode F, Wilcock G. Sexual relationships in married dementia sufferers. Int J Geriatr Psychiatry. 1997;12:447–51.
95. Lochlainn MN, Kenny RA. Sexual activity and aging. J Am Med Dir Assoc. 2013;14:565–72.
96. Wilkins J. More than capacity: alternatives for sexual decision making for individuals with dementia. Gerontologist. 2015;55:717–23.
97. Bauer M, Nay R, Tarzia L, Fetherstonhaugh D, Wellman D, Beattie E, et al. "We need to know what's going on": views of family members toward the sexual expression of people with dementia in residential care. Dementia. 2014;13:571–85.

98. World Health Organization: elder abuse fact sheet, June 2017. Geneva: WHO.

99. Burgess A, Phillips S. Sexual abuse, trauma and dementia in the elderly: a retrospective study of 284 cases. Vict Offenders. 2006;2:193–204.

100. Joy M, Weiss K. Consent for intimacy among persons with neurocognitive impairment. J Am Acad Psychiatry Law. 2018;45:286–94.

101. Graves S. Let's talk about sex: a call for guardianship reform in Washington State. Seattle J Soc Just. 2015;14:477–520.

102. Lyden M. Assessment of sexual consent capacity. Sex Disabil. 2007;25:3–20.

103. Tarzia L, Fetherstonhaugh D, Bauer M. Dementia, sexuality and consent in residential aged care facilities. J Med Ethics. 2012;38:609–13.

104. Abellard J, Rodgers C, Bales A. Balancing sexual expression and risk of harm in elderly persons with dementia. J Am Acad Psychiatry Law. 2017;45:485–92.

105. Lindsay JR. The need for more specific legislation in sexual consent capacity assessments for nursing home residents: how grandpa got his groove back. J Legal Med. 2010;31:303–23.

106. The Society for Post-Acute and Long-Term Care Medicine. White paper: capacity for sexual consent in dementia in long-term care. 2016. Available at https://paltc.org/amda-white-papers-and-resolution-position-statements/capacity-sexual-consent-dementia-long-term-care. Accessed 12 Feb 2018.

107. Cornelison LJ, Doll GM. Management of sexual expression in long-term care: Ombudsmen's perspectives. The Gerontologist. 2012;53(5):780–9.

108. DiNapoli E, Breland GL, Allen RS. Staff knowledge and perceptions of sexuality and dementia of older adults in nursing homes. J Aging Health. 2013;25:1087–105.

109. Gruley B. Sex in geriatrics sets Hebrew Home apart in elderly care. Available at http://www.bloomberg.com/news/print/2013-07-23/sex-in-geriatrics-sets-hebrewhome-apart-in-elderly-care.html. Accessed 12 Feb 2018.

110. Policies and procedures concerning sexual expression at The Hebrew Home at Riverdale. Available at www.hebrewhome.org. Accessed 12 Feb 2018.

111. More J, Marson DC. Assessment of decision-making capacity in older adults: an emerging area of practice and research. J Gerontol. 2007;62(1):3–11.

Chapter 6
Ethical Challenges in Mild, Moderate, and Severe Stages of Dementia

Jananie Kumaran, Rakin Hoq, Romika Dhar, and Meera Balasubramaniam

J. Kumaran
Department of Psychiatry, Saskatchewan Health Authority, Saskatoon, SK, Canada

Department of Psychiatry, Saskatchewan College of Medicine, Saskatoon, SK, Canada
e-mail: jananie.kumaran@saskhealthauthority.ca

R. Hoq
Department of Psychiatry, Summa Health System, Akron, OH, USA
e-mail: hoqr@summahealth.org

R. Dhar
Department of Medicine, West Virginia University School of Medicine, Morgantown, WV, USA
e-mail: romika.dhar@hsc.wvu.edu

M. Balasubramaniam (✉)
New York University School of Medicine, New York, NY, USA
e-mail: meera.balasubramaniam@nyulangone.org

© Springer Nature Switzerland AG 2019
M. Balasubramaniam et al. (eds.), *Psychiatric Ethics in Late-Life Patients*, https://doi.org/10.1007/978-3-030-15172-0_6

Introduction

The population of older adults in the United States is growing at a significant rate. In fact, it is predicted that by the year 2050, the population of individuals aged 65–74 years old will increase from 6% to 9%, and for those who are aged over 75 years, it will increase from 6% to 11% [1]. Dementia is estimated to affect approximately 47 million people worldwide, and it is predicted that by the year 2050, this number will increase to 130 million [1]. Unfortunately, as our population ages, the independence and autonomy of many older adults will be called into question, whether this be due to chronic medical or psychiatric disorders. Older adults are vulnerable to exploitation and abuse due to common cognitive and physical impairments. The changing landscape of increasing life expectancy, advances in the healthcare system, and personal need for autonomy are likely to pose key ethical challenges before individuals, families, and their medical providers. In this chapter, we will use a running case to outline key ethical issues that arise at progressive stages of dementia, following the elegant model adopted by Peter Whitehouse [2]. In the first subsection, we will discuss issues presenting in the early (mild) stages of dementia. These include genetic testing, disclosure of the diagnosis, and the use of cognitive enhancers. This will be followed by discussion of an important issue arising in moderate dementia, namely, the management of behavioral symptoms. Decision-making regarding placement in long-term care facilities will then be described. Finally, issues in end-stage dementia and relevant principles in palliative care will be discussed. For issues on medical decision-making, management of finances, and independent living, readers are referred to the corresponding chapters of this book.

The Case of SR

SR is a 75-year-old man with a medical history of hypertension, coronary artery disease, diabetes, and neuropathy. He has no significant past psychiatric history. He has a family history of Alzheimer's disease on his maternal side. SR works as a mathematics professor at a local university. He has been married for 45 years to his wife and has 3 adult children. SR presents to his primary care physician with his wife with complaints of gradual memory impairment. He states that in the last 1–2 years, he has noticed subtle symptoms, such as forgetting people's names, as well as frequent difficulties in finding his keys and glasses. He describes that more recently; he has been making errors in his classes, resulting in several complaints that have been lodged against him by his students. SR is referred to a cognitive neurologist, and an extensive work up is done, including a neurological exam, comprehensive neurological testing, laboratory tests, and head imaging. He is diagnosed with early stage Alzheimer's disease. SR's wife asks that his physician not inform him of the diagnosis. His daughter contacts the neurologist the following week inquiring if she should consider getting herself tested for susceptibility to Alzheimer's disease.

The diagnosis of mild (early) dementia often brings forth several issues to the table. These include genetic testing, whether or not to disclose the diagnosis of dementia, whether or not to prescribe cognitive enhancers, creating advance care directives, and the need to identify a surrogate decision maker. The last two topics are discussed elsewhere in this book, and therefore will not be discussed in this chapter.

Ethical Issues in Early Stages of Dementia

Genetic Testing

There are four well-established disease-associated genes that have been identified, and numerous chromosomal regions are currently under investigation. The first three well-known genes include 3-APP, PSEN1, and PSEN2 [3]. These three genes represent approximately 3.5% of all cases of Alzheimer's disease. These genes are inherited as autosomal dominant traits, which is linked to the early onset of Alzheimer's disease. Mutations that occur in these genes are deterministic, which means that the affected individual will inevitably develop the disease, if the individual lives long enough. The last established gene associated with disease is ApoE-e4. Mutations of this gene increase the susceptibility to late-onset Alzheimer's disease. Mutations of this gene make up the most common form of this disease [3]. There are some important considerations to make in the discussion of the genetics of Alzheimer's disease. One consideration is predictive genetic testing. In this form of testing, the goal is to predict the future risk of developing Alzheimer's disease in an asymptomatic individual, which is done through the examination of genetic material. This becomes important in the detection of early onset Alzheimer's disease, where family history is negative in 40% of the cases. This is usually due to early death, or failure to recognize the signs in family members. This type of testing is currently restricted to adults from families that show an autosomal dominant pattern with early onset Alzheimer's disease [3]. The second consideration to make is genetic risk assessment. Here, the goal is to identify genetic markers that are known to confer an elevated risk of developing Alzheimer's disease. There is a general consensus that Apo testing has a limited value for predictive testing for Alzheimer's disease in symptomatic people, and therefore the presence of such a marker is neither necessary nor sufficient for the development of Alzheimer's disease [3]. There are opposing arguments as to the merits and demerits of genetic testing. The main merit to this testing would be the ability to prepare for the future. There are several demerits to testing that have been voiced. One is the catastrophic reaction that such testing may bring to the patient and family members. Another demerit is the reality that currently available treatment options have, at best, a modest effect on the disease progression [2]. Finally, there is the possibility of increased healthcare costs, as well as discrimination with employability and insurability. As per the Stanford Program in Genomics, Ethics, and Societies, it is recommended that the "emphasis on development of educational and counseling programs be directed by genetic counselors, informed consent, strict control over the advertising and marketing of genetic tests for Alzheimer's disease, and referral to resources for psychological testing" [2].

Disclosure of Diagnosis

The request from family members to not disclose the diagnosis of Alzheimer's disease to a patient is a common issue encountered in early disease stage. The most commonly cited reasons in the literature that favor not disclosing include the lack of diagnostic certainty, the absence of effective treatments, the potential for adverse psychological reactions, and the inability of persons with developed Alzheimer's disease to understand and/or retain the diagnosis [2]. The most important and obvious reason to inform an individual of the diagnosis of Alzheimer's disease is respect for a patient's autonomy. It is essential if patients are to have an active role in planning for their own care. In the United States and Northern Europe, it is considered best to allow the autonomous individual to have access to this information. In East Asia and Southern Europe, it is considered best to tell the family, and the patient is usually "protected" from the diagnosis [2]. As per the Alzheimer's Association, "As long as a person retains his or her capacity to understand and appreciate the information relevant to a diagnosis, it is important to fully disclose the diagnosis and its implications in a supportive manner" [4]. Early disclosure of diagnosis allows for various decisions. It allows for advanced planning, including the planning for "optimal life experiences in remaining years of intact capacities." It allows for preparing advance directives and power of attorney. It allows for consideration for participation in research. It allows for the participation in support groups. Additionally, it allows for deciding whether to take cognitive enhancers. It has been recommended that disclosure best practices emphasize patient-centered communication techniques in order to minimize psychological distress following diagnosis [2].

Use of Cognitive Enhancers

The use of cognitive enhancers in early stages of illness is often discussed in the geriatric community. Currently, there are four FDA-approved drugs for cognitive enhancers. Rivastigmine, Galantamine, and Donepezil are medications that fall under the class of cholinesterase inhibitors, which are used to improve cognition by inhibiting neuronal acetylcholine breakdown [5]. Memantine is a N-methyl-D-aspartic receptor antagonist, which functions to regulate glutamatergic neurons activities, which facilitates synaptic plasticity, neuronal growth, and differentiation [5, 6]. Currently, the combination of memantine and donepezil is considered the most effective therapy [5, 6]. The use of these FDA-approved medications has been associated with lower rates of dementia progression and cognitive decline in short-term studies. Long-term observational studies have found that persistent use of these medications slows to progression of cognitive, functional, and global decline [5, 6]. Ultimately, the use of these medications delays the need for nursing home placement [6]. Treatment with cognitive enhancers may also reduce total costs of treatment for individuals diagnosed with dementia. For those not treated, there are greater services obtained in hospitals and post-acute care centers, as well as longer length of stays in the hospital. These observations are somewhat offset by the cost in prescriptions, physician visits, and outpatient hospital costs [5, 6]. There are several arguments against the use of these medications. The most important consideration is that these medications provide symptomatic treatment for the disease; however, there is no strong evidence for disease-modifying properties. Another argument relates to the side effects of these medications. The most common side effects include nausea, vomiting, and diarrhea. Less common side effects include anorexia and weight loss, bradycardia, confusion, dizziness, and sleep disturbance [7, 8]. These side effects may present as a safety concern in the prescribing of these medications in the poly-medicated older adult population. Finally, there is a question of tolerability of these medications with relation to quality of life. It is imperative that clinicians engage the patient and families, as applicable, in a comprehensive and careful discussion of the benefits and risks of medications that slow down cognitive decline and help support informed decision-making. For a discussion of advance care directives, readers are directed to the corresponding chapter in this book.

Ethical Issues in Moderate Stages of Dementia

It has been 3 years since SR was diagnosed with Alzheimer's disease. He has just been admitted to the hospital due to paranoia and behavioral issues at home. He believes that his wife has been stealing his money. He has gotten both verbally and physically aggressive toward his wife numerous times, which is a dramatic change from his previous gentle demeanor. In the hospital, SR has refused various forms of treatment, including blood draws and the administration of any medications. SR has undergone psychiatric evaluation, and concluding the evaluation the psychiatrist begins discussing with the family the idea of starting SR on a small dose of quetiapine to target these symptoms. SR's wife is concerned about the idea of "chemically sedating" the psychiatrist and asks if it is truly necessary.

Management of Behavioral Disturbances

As dementia progresses to the mid-stage of disease, cognitive decline becomes more impairing and behavioral issues tend to develop. With progressive deterioration in functioning and decision-making, several ethical issues come into consideration regarding management of the person's health. The most critical issue is the question of a person's capacity to make informed medical decisions regarding their own health. This includes issues of deciding medical treatment, participation in clinical research, and participation in determining the level of care or disposition. This subsection will focus on the ethics of managing behavioral issues associated with dementia using psychotropic medications, in particular, antipsychotic medicines. For a discussion of ethical issues in medical decision-making and participation in research, readers are referred to the corresponding chapters in this book.

Behavioral issues associated with dementia can vary widely, and can include, but are not limited to apathy, depression, mood lability, heightened impulsivity, agitation, paranoia, and even frank psychotic symptoms like hallucinations or delusions. As the disease process progresses, such behavioral symptoms become more frequent and difficult to manage. In fact, up to 50% of people suffering with dementia will at some point experience some degree of psychosis or agitation [9, 10]. It is these symptoms that become the most salient in the management of the illness and raise consideration for use of antipsychotic medications. Both first-generation and second-generation antipsychotics have been studied in the use of managing behavioral issues in dementia. Both classes of medications have demonstrated some benefit in managing symptoms of agitation and psychosis, but large-scale studies and meta-analyses have shown that these benefits are modest overall [11, 12]. These medications are commonly associated with adverse effects, including sedation, extrapyramidal side effects (particularly with the first-generation agents, such as haloperidol), and most concerning-increased risk of cerebrovascular events and death with the second-generation antipsychotics [11,12]. Thus far, there is actually no FDA-approved use for antipsychotic medications in the management of behavioral issues in dementia. The FDA has issued a black box warning against the use of antipsychotics in dementia-related psychosis due to the significantly increased mortality associated with their use [11].

With consideration of the above-stated risks, it is understandable for SR's family to be concerned about the idea of "chemical sedation." It is necessary that as clinicians we recognize and acknowledge such concerns. Perhaps even more importantly, it is imperative that the surrogate decision maker be clearly informed of the risks associated with using these agents since the patient typically cannot make the decision for themselves. Discussion of such risks with these medications is typically quite frightening for families and caregivers, and may deter the consideration of their use. But it is prudent that the clinician frame the potential utility of these medications from both the perspective of the patient's wellbeing and that of the caregivers. In some cases, the administration of antipsychotic medication may be a necessary measure to alleviate the distress of frightening psychotic symptoms, thereby improving the patient's quality of life. In such situations, it becomes imperative to carefully weigh issues of mortality with quality of life. Alternatively, the use of antipsychotic medications may be necessary to manage the patient's aggressive behavior thereby facilitating the viability of the caregiver still being able to care for the patient in their own home. Should these agents be employed in dementia management it is recommended that the lowest effective dose be used to minimize risk of adverse effects.

Ethical Issues in Moderate—End Stages of Dementia

It has been 6 years since SR developed Alzheimer's disease. SR has been experiencing recurrent falls in his home, as well as repeated episodes of urinary tract infections. He has required three hospitalizations this year, each of which has been complicated by delirium. SR was started on quetiapine during one of these hospitalizations due to behavioral disturbances related to delirium. After the third hospitalization, the decision was made to move SR into a nursing home. SR's wife and daughter visit him regularly, though recently he has been withdrawn and has limited interactions. The patient is refusing placement. His family shared emotional challenges and decisional conflicts with respect to nursing home placement.

Placement in a Long-Term Care Facility

As dementia continues to progress, patient needs escalate. New and difficult challenges arise, such as consideration for placement in long-term care facilities and utilization of advance care directives. Advanced care directives will be discussed in depth in the corresponding chapter of this book. For high-income countries, the transition of people with progressive dementia into care homes is a relatively common process, particularly in the last 10 years as the "baby boomer" generation has reached old age [13]. This reflects the high level of care often required for people afflicted by advanced stage dementias. The need for nursing home placement is multifactorial, including issues of medical comorbidity, various psychosocial issues, and neuropsychiatric complications, such as behavioral problems which are focused on in this chapter.

Managing behavioral complications of dementia reaches much further than the bounds of easing the patient's individual experience. Eventually, there comes a point where these symptoms compromise the patient's safety interfere greatly exceed the capabilities of family caretakers. This becomes particularly important in the case of patients who demonstrate wandering behaviors and overt aggression. Behavioral problems in dementia have been consistently shown to be a primary factor associated with caregiver stress [14]. The major conflicting factor with nursing home placement is the idea of separating a person from their own home and family. Patients with mild to moderate dementia have been found to demonstrate awareness of the possibility of future placement and often wish to postpone placement for as long as possible [13]. This raises the ethical dilemma of weighing the patient's own autonomy against the principle of best serving the patient's health needs, i.e. beneficence. But even in more severe cases of dementia when behavioral issues become common and severe, consistency and familiarity of surroundings, routine, and people remain significant factors in preventing behavioral complications [15]. Discussion regarding the need for long-term level of care is, therefore, a critical conversation for clinicians to have with patients' families. As with the discussion of starting antipsychotic medications, it is necessary to frame the conversation of placement from both the perspectives of maintaining autonomy and basic safety. In some cases, such as SR's, nursing home placement may be necessary to meet the needs of a patient's medical comorbidities, or to ensure continued monitoring necessary to maintain safety. But in other cases, separating the patient from their home environment may actually cause unjustified psychological harm and worsening of symptoms.

The autonomy of the patient should be respected as much as possible even in the midst of declining cognition, so determinations of placement should carefully weigh the desires and expectations of both patient and family.

Ethical Issues in End-Stage Dementia

It has been 10 years since SR was diagnosed with Dementia of Alzheimer's type. He has spent the last 4 years in a nursing home. He is now bed bound, has minimal speech output and is completely dependent on nursing care for his ADLs. Family members have raised concerns about SR's declining appetite and weight loss. He has difficulty swallowing and developed pneumonia once this year. They request a consult for feeding tube as they cannot see SR "starve to death". SR does not have a living will on file.

Management of end-stage dementia is complex from both clinical and ethical standpoints. In this section, we will first describe the process of prognostication in dementia. This will be followed by care of commonly encountered end-stage conditions, such as pain, agitation, pneumonia, and weight loss. Identification of distress, empathic communication, and education of families and suitable incorporation of a palliative approach form the cornerstones of good clinical care in end-stage dementia.

Prognostication in Dementia

Dementia is a terminal illness. The long-term prognosis is heterogeneous and variable. However, patients inevitably have a progressive deteriorating course with complications like pneumonia being the most common cause of death. Mean survival time of patients with dementia has been analyzed in cohort studies and case series, ranging from 3 to 11 years [16–18]. The prognosis is determined by the age at diagnosis, gender, and the presence of comorbidities [19]. There are multiple markers of poor short-term survival which include aspiration, recurrent urinary tract infections, pressure ulcers, fever, weight loss, and sepsis. One study found that in nursing home residents with advanced dementia, 6-month mortality for those who developed pneumonia, reduced, eating and fever was 47%, 45%, and 39%, respectively [20]. Not perceiving dementia as a terminal illness can lead to protracted suffering and poor quality of life at end of life. In nursing homes, healthcare professionals have been noted to have overly optimistic prognosis of advanced dementia. A study found that only 1% of patients were perceived to have a life expectancy of less than 6 months but 71% died in that time period [21]. Only 43% of family members perceived dementia as a terminal illness [22]. A US study in nursing home patients with advanced dementia showed that if families had limited understanding of the poor prognosis and clinical course of advanced dementia, patients were more likely to undergo burdensome interventions [23].

Palliative Care in End-Stage Dementia

In contrast to those dying from cancer, those dying from dementia are significantly more likely to receive non-palliative treatments, such as feeding tubes or invasive studies as well as be restrained in the last 30 days of life [21]. As mentioned earlier in this section, prognostication is challenging and many patients can have a "prolonged dwindling" course with severe disability that can persist for years [24]. In the United States, Medicare hospice eligibility criteria for dementia are based on FAST staging [25]. Only patients who are stage 7 with one associated complication (either aspiration, upper urinary tract infection, sepsis, multiple stage 3–4 pressure ulcers, persistent fever, or weight loss of more than 10% in last 6 months) qualify for hospice. However, reliability of the FAST staging is questionable because some patients do not follow a sequential course in FAST.

In 2004, Mitchell et al. developed a 12-item scale which predicted risk of mortality at 6 months in dementia. This scale incorporated an individual's demographic data, comorbidities, such as cancer, heart failure, and the need for oxygen therapy, symptoms like dyspnea, malnutrition data, the presence of intercurrent acute processes, as well as performance data, such as fecal incontinence or bed rest [26]. In 2010, the same researchers revised this scale and published another 12-item prognostic tool: The Advanced Dementia Prognostic Tool (ADEPT) [27] which was consequently validated through a prospective study [28] and found to be superior to the Medicare hospice guidelines in identifying patients with a high risk of death within the next 6 months. The next subsection describes the management of common symptoms encountered in end-stage dementia.

Behavioral problems change qualitatively and quantitatively as dementia progresses. For example, delusions and hallucinations might be less common in the last few months of life, whereas resisting care is more common. Almost any behavioral change is indicative of underlying distress, such as pain, dyspnea, fear, or unmet needs. An optimal approach would be to identify and remove the source of distress. This is best accomplished when multi-disciplinary care teams suitably involve families [15]. Pain is a common cause of suffering and behavioral disturbances in patients with advanced dementia. Due to impaired ability of individuals with dementia to communicate their needs, pain assessment, and management is especially challenging. Nursing home residents with dementia reporting pain are 50% less likely to be treated, when compared to their cognitively preserved counterparts [29]. Hence, observational tools for caregivers that focus on pain associated behaviors like agitation in relation to posture changes and essential personal care, noisy breathing, nonverbal vocalizations (screams and grunts), facial expressions or changes in usual behavior (aggressiveness, refusal to eat, alteration of sleep rhythm, changes in level of activity, etc.) need to be implemented and caregivers need to be educated whether in the community or institutions. As a general rule, it is best to prescribe scheduled analgesics rather than on a needed basis [29].

Autopsy studies have determined that the main causes of death in advanced dementia are pneumonia, cardiovascular diseases, pulmonary embolism, cachexia, and dehydration [30]. When the patients with dementia develop pneumonia, they are commonly hospitalized and treated with antibiotics, primarily parenterally. However, it is important to be aware that the benefits of antibiotic treatment and hospitalization are not well established in this population [31, 32].

Survival after any of these complications is reduced. The burden of hospitalization may far outweigh any benefits. Relevant data must be used to inform and educate families and healthcare professionals, that infection and nutrition problems are to be expected and that their presence usually indicates that the end of the patient's life is near [20]. Weight loss and anorexia are commonly observed in end-stage dementia, and multiple factors such as impaired swallowing reflexes, apraxia, and anosmia contribute to them. One of the most emotionally demanding decisions for families and physicians is the decision about artificial nutrition and hydration. Religious values also determine the beliefs on withholding artificial nutrition. Tube feeding and artificial nutrition may be requested by families due to concerns of their loved one being "starved to death". They often feel they have no choice but to authorize placement of a feeding tube in absence of clear and explicit advanced directives. A study of physicians and nurses found that almost half of them believed that even if all forms of life support are stopped, nutrition and hydration should be continued [33].

As many as 44% of nursing home residents with advanced dementia have feeding tubes placed [34]. There is compelling evidence that artificial feeding does not improve life expectancy or quality of life, nor does it prevent aspiration pneumonia in advanced dementia [35]. When tube feeding is used as permanent substitute to oral feeding, patients are deprived of the pleasure derived from eating. The most serious consequence of tube feeding is the need to restrain some patients. Peck et al. observed that a whopping 71% patients with dementia who had feeding tubes had been restrained [36]. Growing literature from hospice settings indicates that patients in end stages of dementia do not experience more than transient hunger and thirst which can be alleviated with the use of ice chips and mouth swabs [37].

Defining optimal palliative care in dementia has been a focus of research and development by multiple experts. In 2014, the European association for palliative care published a framework to provide guidance for clinical practice, policy, and research. This framework covers aspects such improving quality of life, maintaining functioning, and maximizing comfort throughout the disease trajectory, adequate treatment of behavioral and psychological symptoms of dementia, comorbid diseases and inter or concurrent health problems, person-centered care, communication and shared decision-making, proactively setting care goals and advance planning, prognostication and timely recognition of dying, avoidance of overtly aggressive, burdensome and futile treatments, provision of psychosocial and spiritual support, education of the healthcare team, and societal and ethical issues [38]. In the United States, the use of hospice services for end-stage dementia has increased from 19.3% to 48% from 2000 to 2009, which is an encouraging trend. However, a vast majority of patients continue to be hospitalized in their last 90 days of life leading to burdensome interventions, and multiple transitions of care [39]. The use of hospice is associated with improved patient and caregiver outcomes, improved pain management, less aggressive care, and greater satisfaction among family members [40].

Conclusion

Dementia brings to the table, numerous ethical challenges at every stage of the illness. It is imperative that clinicians consistently emphasize on a model of care that is patient-centered, even when an individual with dementia become less capable of communicating one's needs. Toward this, one must engage in regular and timely communication, education of patients and families, and engage them empathically in a process of shared decision-making. Research focusing on ethical issues in dementia must encompass not only clinical outcomes but also subjective experiences of patients and families.

References

1. Alzheimer's Disease International. World Alzheimer Report 2015. https://www.alz.co.uk/research/world-report-2015. Accessed 18 Apr 2018.
2. Whitehouse P. Ethical issues in dementia. Dialogues Clin Neurosci. 2000;2:162–7.
3. Leuzy A, Gauthier S. Ethical issues in Alzheimer's disease: an overview. Expert Rev Neurother. 2012;12(5):557–67.
4. Alzheimer's Association. https://www.alz.org/. Accessed 18 Apr 2018.
5. Rountree SD, Atri A, Lopez OL, Doody RS. Effectiveness of antidementia drugs in delaying Alzheimer's disease progression. Alzheimers Dement. 2013;9(3):338–45.
6. Fillit H, Hill J. Economics of dementia and pharmacoeconomics of dementia therapy. Am J Geriatr Pharmacother. 2005;3(1):39–49.
7. Tampi R, Tampi D, Lavakumar M. Pharmacology and psychopharmacology. In: Rajesh R, Tampi D, Boyle L. Psychiatric disorders late in life, A comprehensive review. New York: Springer; 2018. p. 279.
8. Pataki C, Sussman N. Psychopharmacological treatments- cholinesterase inhibitors and memantine. In: Sadock B, Sadock V, Ruiz P. Synopsis of psychiatry. Wolters Kluwer; 2015. p. 963–4.
9. Treloar A, Crugel M, Prasanna A, Solomons L, Fox C, Paton C, et al. Ethical dilemmas: should antipsychotics ever be prescribed for people with dementia? Br J Psychiatry. 2010;197(02):88–90.
10. Jeste DV, Finkel SI. Psychosis of Alzheimers disease and related dementias: diagnostic criteria for a distinct syndrome. Am J Geriatr Psychiatry. 2000;8(1):29–34.
11. Schneider LS, Tariot PN, Dagerman KS, Davis SM, Hsiao JK, Ismail S, et al. Effectiveness of atypical antipsychotic drugs in patients with Alzheimer's disease. N Engl J Med. 2006;355(4):416–8.
12. Sink KM, Holden KF, Yaffe K. Pharmacological treatment of neuropsychiatric symptoms of dementia. JAMA. 2005;293(5):596–608.
13. Smebye KL, Kirkevold M, Engedal K. Ethical dilemmas concerning autonomy when persons with dementia wish to live at home: a qualitative, hermeneutic study. BMC Health Serv Res. 2015;16(1):21.

14. Sörensen S, Conwell Y. Issues in dementia caregiving: effects on mental and physical health, intervention strategies, and research needs. Am J Geriatr Psychiatry. 2011;19(6):491–6.
15. Kales HC, Gitlin LN, Lyketsos CG. Assessment and management of behavioral and psychological symptoms of dementia. BMJ. 2015;350:h369.
16. Fitzpatrick AL, Kuller LH, Lopez OL, Kawas CH, Jagust W. Survival following dementia onset: Alzheimer's disease and vascular dementia. J Neurol Sci. 2005;229–230:43–9.
17. Dewey ME, Saz P. Dementia, cognitive impairment and mortality in persons aged 65 and over living in the community: a systematic review of the literature. Int J Geriatr Psychiatry. 2001;16(8):751–61.
18. Knopman DS, Rocca WA, Cha RH, Edland SD, Kokmen E. Survival study of vascular dementia in Rochester, Minnesota. Arch Neurol. 2003;60(1):85–90.
19. Xie J, Brayne C, Matthews FE, Medical Research Council Cognitive Function and Ageing Study Collaborators. Survival times in people with dementia: analysis from population based cohort study with 14-year follow-up. BMJ. 2008;336(7638):258–62.
20. Mitchell SL, Teno JM, Kiely DK, Shaffer ML, Jones RN, Prigerson HG, et al. The clinical course of advanced dementia. N Engl J Med. 2009;361(16):1529–38.
21. Mitchell SL, Kiely DK, Hamel MB. Dying with advanced dementia in the nursing home. Arch Intern Med. 2004;164:321–6.
22. van der Steen JT, Onwuteaka-Philipsen BD, Knol DL, Ribbe MW, Deliens L. Caregivers' understanding of dementia predicts patients' comfort at death: a prospective observational study. BMC Med. 2013;11:105.
23. Caron C, Griffith J, Arcand M. Decision making at the end of life in dementia: how family caregivers perceive their interactions with health care providers in long-term- care settings. J Appl Gerontol. 2005;24:231–47.
24. Lunney JR, Lynn J, Foley DJ, Lipson S, Guralnik JM. Patterns of functional decline at the end of life. JAMA. 2003;289(18):2387–92.
25. Reisberg B. Functional assessment staging (FAST). Psychopharmacol Bull. 1988;24:653–9.
26. Mitchell SL, Kiely DK, Hamel MB, Park PS, Morris JN, Fries BE. Estimating prognosis for nursing home residents with advanced dementia. JAMA. 2004;291(22):2734–40.
27. Mitchell SL, Miller SC, Teno JM, Davis RB, Shaffer ML. The advanced dementia prognostic tool: a risk score to estimate

survival in nursing home residents with advanced dementia. J Pain Symptom Manag. 2010;40(5):639–51.

28. Mitchell SL, Miller SC, Teno JM, Kiely DK, Davis RB, Shaffer ML. Prediction of 6-month survival of nursing home residents with advanced dementia using ADEPT vs hospice eligibility guidelines. JAMA. 2010;304(17):1929–35.

29. Won A, Lapane K, Gambassi G, Bernabei R, Mor V, Lipsitz LA. Correlates and management of nonmalignant pain in the nursing home. J Am Geriatr Soc. 1999;47:936–42.

30. Keene J. Death and dementia. Int J Geriatr Psychiatry. 2001;16(10):969–74.

31. Van der Steen JT, Ooms ME, van der Wal G, Ribbe MW. Pneumonia: the demented patient's best friend? Discomfort after starting or withholding antibiotic treatment. J Am Geriatr Soc. 2002;50(10):1681–8.

32. Van der Steen JT, Ooms ME, van der Wal G, Ribbe MW. Withholding or starting antibiotic treatment in patients with dementia and pneumonia: prediction of mortality with physicians' judgment of illness severity and with specific prognostic models. Med Decis Mak. 2005;25(2):210–21.

33. Solomon MZ, O'Donnell L, Jennings B, Guilfoy V, Wolf SM, Nolan K, et al. Decisions near the end of life: professional views on life-sustaining treatments. Am J Public Health. 1993;83(1):14–23.

34. Teno JM, Mor V, Desilva D, Kabumoto G, Roy J, Wetle T. Use of feeding tubes in nursing home residents with severe cognitive impairment. JAMA. 2002;287:3211–2.

35. Finucane TE, Christmas C, Travis K. Tube feeding in patients with advanced dementia. JAMA. 1999;282:1365–70.

36. Peck A, Cohen CE, Mulvihill MN. Long-term enteral feeding of aged demented nursing home patients. J Am Geriatr Soc. 1990;38(11):1195–8.

37. McCann RM, Hall WJ, Groth-Junker A. Comfort care for terminally ill patients: the appropriate use of nutrition and hydration. JAMA. 1994;272(16):1263–6.

38. Van der Steen JT, Radbruch L, Hertogh CM, de Boer ME, Hughes JC, Larkin P, et al. White paper defining optimal palliative care in older people with dementia: a Delphi study and recommendations from the European Association for Palliative Care. Palliat Med. 2014;28(3):197–209.

39. Teno JM, Gozalo PL, Bynum JP, Leland NE, Miller SC, Morden NE, et al. Change in end-of-life care for Medicare beneficiaries:

site of death, place of care, and health care transitions in 2000, 2005, and 2009. JAMA. 2013;309(5):470–7.

40. Shega JW, Hougham GW, Stocking CB, Cox-Hayley D, Sachs GA. Patients dying with dementia: experience at the end of life and impact of hospice care. J Pain Symptom Manag. 2008;35(5):499–507.

Chapter 7
Research Ethics
in Geriatric Psychiatry

Laura B. Dunn and Iuliana Predescu

Introduction

Research gaps outnumber what is known about the treatment of psychiatric disorders in late life. The increase in the population of older adults with psychiatric and neurocognitive disorders, and the relative lack of evidence-based treatments for their symptoms and syndromes, argue strongly for an ongoing research imperative—i.e., for basic, translational, and clinical investigations focused on psychiatric and neurocognitive disorders of late life. These studies will require human volunteers, including those with and without specific disorders, to participate in research. In some cases, the studies might benefit the volunteers directly; however, in many if not most cases, the only beneficiaries are science and—hopefully—future patients.

Moreover, as neuroscience research makes forays into increasingly innovative territory (e.g., responsive neuromodulation, brain-machine interfaces), and as research frameworks

L. B. Dunn (✉)
Department of Psychiatry and Behavioral Sciences,
Stanford University, Stanford, CA, USA
e-mail: laura.dunn@stanford.edu

I. Predescu
UPMC Altoona, Altoona, PA, USA
e-mail: predescui@upmc.edu

© Springer Nature Switzerland AG 2019   109
M. Balasubramaniam et al. (eds.), *Psychiatric Ethics in Late-Life Patients*, https://doi.org/10.1007/978-3-030-15172-0_7

evolve — leading to the possibility of earlier and earlier prediction of neurocognitive disorders (e.g., preclinical Alzheimer's disease [AD]) — the array of ethical issues confronting researchers as well as clinicians will expand.

Ethical considerations in research with older populations arise at all stages of the research endeavor, from conceptualization of the research question, to study design, to recruitment and retention, to the actual study conduct itself, to analysis of results, and dissemination of findings. Research ethics encompasses a broad range of topics — e.g., informed consent, decision-making capacity and its assessment, surrogate consent, investigator conflicts of interest, and institutional review board (IRB)/research ethics committee review, approval, and oversight. For the purposes of this chapter, however, we will focus only on a few of these topics, i.e., informed consent, decision-making capacity, and surrogate consent to research, as these topics have been the subject of substantial empirical ethics study.

Informed Consent for Research

The pillars of ethical research conduct have been outlined in numerous important codes, declarations, and documents over the last 70-plus years — including the Nuremberg Code, the Declaration of Helsinki, and The Belmont Report (for a more detailed review of important documents in the history of research ethics, see [1]). In the United States, the Belmont Report (formally titled, "Ethical Principles and Guidelines for the Protection of Human Subjects of Research") laid out three broad principles for the ethical conduct of research [2]. The Report also very usefully discussed the operationalization of these principles (i.e., via informed consent, analysis of risks and benefits, and appropriate subject selection). Further, the Report illustrates how the three principles may exist in tension in the research context, acknowledging in plain language that there are not always simple solutions to complex issues that arise in research. In other words, the Report is not a list of hard-and-fast rules, or a checklist to be followed, but rather is meant to serve as a guide to thoughtful deliberation and decision-making by researchers and reviewers. In this sense, the Belmont Report has been an extremely important document in the field of research ethics. The three principles, as defined in the Belmont Report, are as follows:

- *"Respect for persons: Respect for persons incorporates at least two ethical convictions: first, that individuals should be treated as autonomous agents, and second, that persons with diminished autonomy are entitled to protection. The principle of respect for persons thus divides into two separate moral requirements: the requirement to acknowledge autonomy and the requirement to protect those with diminished autonomy."*
- *"Beneficence: Persons are treated in an ethical manner not only by respecting their decisions and protecting them from harm, but also by making efforts to secure their well-being…. Two general rules have been formulated as complementary expressions of beneficent actions in this sense: (1) do not harm and (2) maximize possible benefits and minimize possible harms."*
- *"Justice: Who ought to receive the benefits of research and bear its burdens? This is a question of justice, in the sense of 'fairness in distribution' or 'what is deserved'. An injustice occurs when some benefit to which a person is entitled is denied without good reason or when some burden is imposed unduly"* [2].

Informed consent flows directly from the first principle, respect for persons, as it mandates respecting the autonomy of individuals, operationalized in their willing and informed decision-making. In circumstances where informed consent by the potential participant is not possible (e.g., advanced dementia), the protection of the individual with diminished autonomy takes precedence, as discussed in the section on Surrogate Consent.

As has been discussed in detail elsewhere [3], informed consent for research is generally viewed as consisting of three required components: (1) disclosure of information relevant to the research decision, i.e., the purpose, nature, and procedures of the study; study risks, benefits, and alternatives; (2) decision-making capacity; and (3) voluntariness (a free and genuine choice made without of coercion) [4].

Decision-making capacity itself has been sub-divided into four requisite abilities, namely (1) understanding, i.e., adequate comprehension of relevant information; (2) appreciation, i.e., the ability to grasp how the research-related information applies to one's own circumstances; (3) reasoning, i.e., abilities to weigh information and reason through the consequences of one's decision; and (4) choice, i.e., the ability to communicate a clear and consistent choice—in the case of research, this amounts to a stable decision regarding participation [3]. It should be noted that this model of decision-making capacity is just that—a model meant to serve as a guide for covering key aspects of the decision at hand. Although there are several instruments available to aid in capacity assessment, there remains no true "gold standard" for assessing capacity [5]. Furthermore, reasonable physicians can come to different conclusions about whether a patient possesses or lacks capacity for a specific task. Importantly, most experts would argue that the standard for capacity should vary depending on the nature of the decision, i.e., a sliding scale should be used wherein higher-stakes decisions require a higher threshold of capacity. In general, because of the relative lack of consensus regarding tools and cut-points, we do not recommend a specific cut-point on a specific capacity assessment tool. However, investigators should consult with their local Institutional Review Board/Research Ethics Committee (IRB/REC) to ensure that appropriate capacity assessments are incorporated into their research protocols when needed. Of note, there is also no consistent regulatory guidance about this aspect of psychiatric research; in the United States, only a few states, for example, have specific laws related to assigning a surrogate for consent for research [6].

It should be noted, though, that numerous studies examining capacity to consent to research among people with a variety of psychiatric disorders have demonstrated that, while the majority of adults with psychiatric disorders retain the requisite abilities to provide informed consent for research, there is substantial heterogeneity among this population. In other words, some individuals with mental illness are vulnerable to impaired decision-making capacity; these impairments tend to be associated with cognitive deficits rather than with psychiatric symptoms per se [7].

It follows, then, that when older adults who may have cognitive impairment (regardless of underlying etiology) are being considered as potential research participants, additional safeguards around informed consent are likely needed. Such safeguards may include capacity screening, use of enhanced consent procedures, or inclusion of a study "partner" (an individual, often a relative of the patient, who is involved in the consent process and study visits) or subject advocate [8, 9].

Surrogate Consent

In studying geriatric patients with a known diagnosis of a neurodegenerative disorder such as AD or other forms of dementia, investigators inevitably must grapple with the issue of determining how they will ethically enroll these participants. In most cases, ethical research conduct will require obtaining informed consent from someone other than the patient, as well as obtaining "assent" from the patient him/herself. The person providing informed consent on behalf of the patient is variously referred to as the patient's surrogate, proxy, alternate decision-maker, or legally authorized representative (with the caveat that the latter term can be confusing when the law is silent on who is legally authorized to make research decisions on behalf of the patient).

The reality is that in neurodegenerative disorders, patients inevitably lose decisional capacity during the course of the illness. One of the more challenging issues has been determining when this loss of capacity tends to occur. In studies that used detailed capacity assessment tools (e.g., the MacArthur Competence Assessment Tool for Clinical Research), the consistent finding has been that most patients lose capacity at some point during the transition from mild to moderate AD [10–12]. However, given the move to a biologically defined research framework for AD [13], further research will be needed to determine how the new biologically defined categories of disease relate to levels of capacity, as well as whether certain disease characteristics correspond to specific decisional deficits.

Although surrogate consent is widely used in dementia research, relatively little is known about the nature of surrogates' decision-making processes, i.e., how they make a decision on behalf of their loved one. The ethics literature (as well as a few state laws) emphasize that surrogate decision-makers should make a decision using a "substituted judgment" standard (i.e., stepping into the decisionally incapable person's shoes to make a decision based on how that person would have decided). However, it is not apparent that this is actually how surrogates make these decisions. In a study of surrogate decision-makers for people with AD (who were given a hypothetical clinical trial protocol and asked to discuss whether and why they would enroll their relative), surrogates described using both substituted judgment as well as considering the patient's best interests [14]. Essentially, these surrogates were engaged in a balancing act—trying to honor (their perception of the) patient's wishes and abiding values while simultaneously striving to maintain the patient's quality of life. For example, one participant described trying to consider the type of person her mother was, as well as the potential risks of the study:

> Now with her, you have to take into consideration what kind of person she is to begin with. Then you have to think about, at this age, do you subject somebody to any unnecessary risk? And you have to evaluate…well, the trade-off. Is the likelihood of benefiting science large enough to offset the likelihood of her inconvenience and her discomfort? It's very different when you're thinking about it for somebody else than for yourself [14].

It is not even clear that cognitively impaired individuals and their surrogate decision-makers actually perceive the decision process similarly. For example, Black and colleagues interviewed research pairs (cognitively impaired adults and their surrogates), asking them about the process they had used when deciding to enroll in a research study (in this case, a study they had actually participated in). Frequent disagreement was noted between the surrogate and the cognitively impaired individual regarding how the decision was made [15]. Several other studies found that surrogates' decisions about research appeared to more closely track their own preferences as opposed to those of the patient [16, 17].

When asked specifically about their motivations for enrolling their relative with dementia in research, surrogate decision-makers have cited the following reasons: potential for direct benefit to the patient; altruism or benefits in the future to others; medical evaluation/diagnostic procedures; compensation; attention from research staff/clinicians; access to more precise treatment; trust in researchers/research; and educational value [18].

The potential for overestimation of direct benefit remains a problem in clinical research, including research focusing on dementia. In some instances, this overestimation may stem from difficulty understanding that clinical research is not the same as standard-of-care treatment. While less studied so far in dementia research, concerns about the "therapeutic misconception" (a failure to appreciate key distinctions between research and treatment) have been raised in clinical research generally [19–21].

Clearly describing for potential subjects and their family members the purpose of the research, as well as (when applicable) the limits of what is currently known about the treatment being studied, may help mitigate this sort of misunderstanding. Nancy King, in an effort to reduce misplaced optimism about direct benefits of research for participants, argued for a more clear-cut delineation of types of potential benefit in trials, i.e. [22],

- *Direct benefit, …properly defined as benefit arising from receiving the intervention being studied*

- *Collateral benefit to subjects …benefit arising from being a subject, even if one does not receive the experimental intervention (e.g., a free physical examination and testing, free medical care and other extras, or personal gratification of altruism)*
- *Aspirational benefit, or benefit to society and to future patients, which arises from the results of the study* [22]

Whether such description of benefits in consent forms and discussions would help participants better appreciate the nature and likelihood of benefit in dementia research is, thus far, unclear.

Future Directions

Geriatric psychiatry deals with some of the most difficult-to-treat conditions in medicine. Ethical enrollment of older adults with a wide range of psychiatric and cognitive disorders will remain of paramount importance for the knowledge base to advance. Numerous issues related to the ethics of research involving older adults with psychiatric and cognitive disorders remain understudied and unaddressed. These include the following:

- Legal and policy issues—e.g., the legal status of research on individuals with diminished capacity due to neurocognitive disorders; legal and regulatory guidance regarding surrogate consent for research
- Empirical questions about decision-making capacity—e.g., when is it appropriate or necessary to conduct formal capacity assessment; what tools should be used to conduct such assessments; who should do these assessments; where should the line be drawn between adequate and impaired capacity; and how should this line vary depending on the nature of the research?
- Surrogate consent issues—e.g., how best to engage surrogates in the consent process; when and how to assess surrogates' own understanding of research; how to evaluate

whether surrogates are weighing the risks and benefits of research appropriately for the patient?
- Review and oversight issues—e.g., how should IRBs define and weigh risks and benefits in considering research involving individuals with diminished capacity.

Conclusions

Geriatric psychiatry research will become increasingly needed in an era of major demographic shifts to an aging population. While we have attempted to provide an overview of some of the ethical issues that arise in the conduct of research with older adults, undoubtedly there are additional issues that are likely to emerge. Investigators who are conducting—or hope to conduct—research involving older adults and their families need to be versed in the ethical foundations of human subjects research, including past history of abuses and exploitation particularly involving vulnerable populations such as people with mental illness. The "research imperative" can be met while also meeting our ethical obligations to participants, but this requires ongoing vigilance regarding the ethics of research, as well as the humility to acknowledge how much we do not know about the human brain, as well as human motivations. Research on the ethics of research is also needed to continue to flesh out these important issues, particularly as research on the brain moves into ever more technologically sophisticated realms.

References

1. Fischer BA. A summary of important documents in the field of research ethics. Schizophr Bull. 2006;32:69–80.
2. National Commission for the Protection of Human Subjects of Biomedical and Behavioral Research. The Belmont report: ethical principles and guidelines for the protection of human subjects of research. Washington, DC: Government Printing Office; 1979.

3. Appelbaum PS, Grisso T. MacCAT-CR: MacArthur competence assessment tool for clinical research. Sarasota: Professional Resource Press; 2001.
4. Faden RR, Beauchamp TL, King NMP. A history and theory of informed consent. New York: Oxford University Press; 1986.
5. Dunn LB, Nowrangi MA, Palmer BW, Jeste DV, Saks ER. Assessing decisional capacity for clinical research or treatment: a review of instruments. Am J Psychiatry. 2006;163:1323–34.
6. DeMartino ES, Dudzinski DM, Doyle CK, Sperry BP, Gregory SE, Siegler M, et al. Who decides when a patient can't? Statutes on alternate decision makers. N Engl J Med. 2017;376:1478–82.
7. Dunn LB, Candilis PJ, Roberts LW. Emerging empirical evidence on the ethics of schizophrenia research. Schizophr Bull. 2006;32:47–68.
8. Stroup TS, Appelbaum PS. Evaluation of a "subject advocate" in the Clinical Antipsychotic Trials of Intervention Effectiveness (CATIE) schizophrenia study. Schizophr Bull. 2006;32:147–52.
9. Stroup S, Appelbaum P. The subject advocate: protecting the interests of participants with fluctuating decisionmaking capacity. IRB. 2003;25:9–11.
10. Kim SY, Caine ED, Currier GW, Leibovici A, Ryan JM. Assessing the competence of persons with Alzheimer's disease in providing informed consent for participation in research. Am J Psychiatry. 2001;158:712–7.
11. Kim SY, Caine ED. Utility and limits of the mini mental state examination in evaluating consent capacity in Alzheimer's disease. Psychiatr Serv. 2002;53:1322–4.
12. Kim SY, Karlawish JH. Ethics and politics of research involving subjects with impaired decision-making abilities. Neurology. 2003;61:1645–6.
13. Jack CR Jr, Bennett DA, Blennow K, Carrillo MC, Dunn B, Haeberlein SB, et al. NIA-AA research framework: toward a biological definition of Alzheimer's disease. Alzheimers Dement. 2018;14:535–62.
14. Dunn LB, Fisher SR, Hantke M, Appelbaum PS, Dohan D, Young JP, et al. "Thinking about it for somebody else": Alzheimer's disease research and proxy decision makers' translation of ethical principles into practice. Am J Geriatr Psychiatry. 2013;21:337–45.
15. Black BS, Wechsler M, Fogarty L. Decision making for participation in dementia research. Am J Geriatr Psychiatry. 2013;21:355–63.

16. Sachs GA, Stocking CB, Stern R, Cox DM, Hougham G, Sachs RS. Ethical aspects of dementia research: informed consent and proxy consent. Clin Res. 1994;42:403–12.

17. Hougham GW, Sachs GA, Danner D, Mintz J, Patterson M, Roberts LW, et al. Empirical research on informed consent with the cognitively impaired. IRB. 2003;Suppl 25:S26–32.

18. Dunn LB, Hoop JG, Misra S, Fisher SR, Roberts LW. "A feeling that you're helping": proxy decision making for Alzheimer's research. Narrat Inq Bioeth. 2011;1:107–22.

19. Appelbaum PS, Lidz CW, Grisso T. Therapeutic misconception in clinical research: frequency and risk factors. IRB. 2004;26:1–8.

20. Lidz CW, Albert K, Appelbaum P, Dunn LB, Overton E, Pivovarova E. Why is therapeutic misconception so prevalent? Camb Q Healthc Ethics. 2015;24:231–41.

21. Lidz CW, Appelbaum PS. The therapeutic misconception: problems and solutions. Med Care. 2002;40(9 Suppl):V55–63.

22. King NM. Defining and describing benefit appropriately in clinical trials. J Law Med Ethics. 2000;28:332–43.

Part II
Medicolegal Aspects
of Geriatric Psychiatry

Chapter 8
Advance Healthcare Planning

Aarti Gupta and Romika Dhar

Introduction

As life expectancy has increased over the last century, so has the length of life lived with diseases and illnesses [1, 2]. Advances in the medical field have made a wide array of treatments and services available for terminal illnesses, ranging from aggressive invasive procedures to comfort measures and palliative care. Although healthcare providers and family members often find it compelling to implement life-saving measures, some of these procedures can severely compromise quality of life and cause unnecessary sufferings to individuals at the end of their life.

A. Gupta (✉)
Yale University School of Medicine, New Haven, CT, USA
e-mail: aarti.gupta@yale.edu

R. Dhar
Department of Medicine, West Virginia University School of Medicine, Morgantown, WV, USA
e-mail: romika.dhar@hsc.wvu.edu

© Springer Nature Switzerland AG 2019   123
M. Balasubramaniam et al. (eds.), *Psychiatric Ethics in Late-Life Patients*, https://doi.org/10.1007/978-3-030-15172-0_8

Clinical evidence indicates that aggressive procedures do not always translate into better quality of life, and contrary to the seemingly obvious option, life-prolonging measures are not always an individual's preference.

Older adults are at an increased risk for losing decision-making capacity due to many conditions common to old age, making it difficult for them to make their treatment choices known when they need to. In an event that the older adults lose their decision-making capacity, and if their wishes for treatments are not known, then they may receive treatments that they may not have chosen for themselves had they been able to state their preferences. Advance healthcare planning can help older adults make treatment choices in advance of losing decisional capacity and to receive care in keeping with their wishes, goals, and values. Advance healthcare planning is a process whereby individuals, in consultation with their healthcare providers, family members, and important others make decisions about his or her future health care in order to prepare for future medical care decisions should a time come when they are unable to make such decisions [3].

A Brief History

Advance healthcare planning, as it is known today, has undergone many changes and iterations over the years [4–6]. The concept of "Living Will," a tool through which individuals could state their wishes about future treatments was first proposed by a Chicago-based human rights lawyer, Luis Kutner in 1967. This proposal resulted in a simple form being developed by the Euthanasia Society of America in 1972, which stated that if an individual did not have a reasonable chance of recovery from medical illnesses, they were allowed to die, if they so wished. The Living Will concept gained a major impetus in 1975 with the case of Karen Ann Quinlan, a 21-year-old woman, who suffered brain damage and was declared to be in a persistent vegetative state at a New Jersey (NJ) hospital. Her parents requested the hospital to discontinue the ventilator but were turned down, a decision also upheld by the NJ superior court. The Quinlans then appealed the case in the NJ Supreme Court, who granted their request. Ms. Quinlan surprisingly continued to breathe after being taken off of the respirator and died 9 years later in 1985 at a nursing home from respiratory failure. Following Quinlan's case, California passed the Natural Death Act in 1976, which allowed competent adults to refuse life-sustaining treatment for incurable injury or illness, and sanctioned the first Living Will. Many states followed suit and currently all states have some version of the Living Will.

Advance healthcare planning saw another landmark development in the first "right to die" case of Nancy Cruzan in 1983 [7]. Nancy Cruzan was a 23-year-old woman who ended up in a persistent vegetative state following a motor vehicle accident. She was in need of total care and tube feedings and after hoping for recovery for several years, her parents asked for her tube feeds to be stopped. The rehabilitation facility refused, until her parents got a court order from the US Supreme Court, after initially losing their case in the Missouri Supreme court. The Supreme Court acknowledged the right of an individual to die, but rested the final version of those statutes in the hands of the state. The case went back to Missouri Supreme court, which required the Cruzans to prove that Nancy would not have wanted to live under these circumstances. Her family and friends shared information with court about their conversation with Nancy about quality and end of life that they had in years prior. In 1990, all feeding tubes were removed leading to her demise. The Congress passed the 1990 Patient Self Determination Act in response to Nancy Cruzan case as a part of Omnibus Budget Reconciliation Act (OBRA). It underwent a few revisions and the way it stands today, it mandates Medicaid and Medicare provider organizations to give information to patients about advance directives (ADs) and their right to formulate those in writing upon admission.

Patient Self Determination Act of 1990 [8, 9] amends titles XVIII (Medicare) and XIX (Medicaid) of the Social Security Act to require hospitals, skilled nursing facilities, home health agencies, hospice programs, and health maintenance organizations to (1) inform patients of their rights under State law to make decisions concerning their medical care; (2) periodically inquire as to whether a patient executed an advanced directive and document the patient's wishes regarding their medical care; (3) not discriminate against persons who have executed an advance directive; (4) ensure that legally valid advance directives and documented medical care wishes are implemented to the extent permitted by State law; and (5) provide educational programs for staff, patients, and the community on ethical issues concerning patient self-determination and advance directives.

There have been many more developments since these landmark cases (Table 8.1). In one of the most recent impor-

TABLE 8.1 Evolution of advance healthcare planning and advance directives [7–10]

Year	Developments
1967	1st Advance Directives proposed by Euthanasia Society of America representative, Luis Kutner
1975	NJ Supreme Court grants order to discontinue ventilator in Karen Ann Quinlan case
1976	California becomes the first state to sanction the Living Will in the form of the Natural Death Act
1983	California adopts first Power of Attorney (PoA) for healthcare
1990	US Supreme Court allows discontinuation of tube feeds in Nancy Cruzan case in the first ever "right to die" case
1990	Creation of the advance healthcare directives through approval of Patient Self Determination Act in response to Nancy Cruzan case
1991	Physician Orders for Life-Sustaining Treatment (POLST) paradigm begins in Oregon
By 1999	Discussions about implementing Do-Not-Resuscitate (DNR) orders leading to 42 states adopting the DNR protocols
By 2009	44 states and District of Columbia have some version of default surrogate laws
2016	Medicare allows one doctor patient session to discuss end-of-life issues

tant developments, the Centers for Medicare and Medicaid Services (CMS), finalized regulations that allow Medicare to pay clinicians and other qualified healthcare professionals for providing advance care planning consultation to beneficiaries from January 2016 [10].

The Process of Advance Healthcare Planning

Advance healthcare planning involves many steps from initiation to their implementation. Although it can be started at any age or stage of a disease process; most often, these conversations start once a person receives a terminal diagnosis. It is important that advance healthcare planning commences as soon as possible with older adults while they are still healthy and able to collaborate in choosing their treatment options and stating their choices. If an individual does not seem receptive to having a conversation regarding advance healthcare planning, the clinician should assess and address the barriers to these communications. Involving a loved one and inviting them to these discussions helps facilitate these difficult conversations by encouraging collaboration and providing support to the individual. If a surrogate decision-maker has not been chosen, it should be encouraged during this process, as it helps surrogates feel more comfortable in their role and reduces the distress from such critical decision-making in the future.

The most crucial element of this process is to get an understanding of the patient's values and beliefs that will guide their treatment choices and decision-making [11, 12]. The importance of face-to-face communication between the clinician, the patient, and preferably their loved one in this process cannot be overstated [13]. A meta-analysis indicated that the use of structured communication tools like the "Values History" as opposed to ad-hoc approaches may increase the frequency of discussions about, and completion of, advance directives and the concordance between the care that is desired and finally received by patients [14]. Values History is a two-part form that allows patients to identify their values and beliefs regarding terminal care in first part and makes provision to complete advance directives in the second part [15].

Advance healthcare planning is not a one-time event but a process that should ideally include ongoing discussions that not only enhance the clinician's understanding of patient's care goals but also give the patient a chance to evolve their own formulation of the plan and make informed decisions. The healthcare plan may have to go through several iterations and changes with changes in patient's disease process or circumstances. Incorporating patient's wishes in ongoing care helps everyone understand their treatment choices better.

Advance Directives

Advance healthcare planning is formalized into a legal document called advance directives, which is a key instrument in helping the execution of healthcare planning. Different states vary in their law statutes governing advance directives and forms. Clinicians and patients must therefore familiarize themselves with these procedures specific to their state before starting the process.

There are two different forms of advance directives [16], although an individual can formulate one document with the elements of both [17]:

1. Living Will
2. Power of Attorney

A Living Will is a document that gives directives to clinicians and surrogate decision-makers regarding the treatment that a person may or may not want at the end of life [18]. It includes items such as life-sustaining treatments including resuscitation, intubation, tube feeding, dialysis, medication preferences (e.g., chemotherapy), and organ and tissue donation. It may also document the individual's wishes in regards to palliative care management including pain management, invasive tests, and procedures (e.g., implanting a defibrillator) and where the person wishes to die. Generally, Living Will goes into effect when a person is diagnosed with a condition specified in their state's Living Will law and when two different clinicians certify patient's loss of capacity, but these specifics vary widely from state to state.

Living Will is based on predicting possible future medical scenarios and addressing those ahead of time. However, real-life situations are more complex than what could be addressed through Living Will, which has led to the formulation of a Power of Attorney. Simply put, a Power of Attorney is a legal document wherein a person gives another person the right and the power to act on their behalf. The person (referred to as the "principal") may choose to vest very specific powers in another person (referred to as the "agent") in matters of private affairs, business, or other legal matters, e.g., allowing the agent to manage their finance if they were out of country. An important consideration is that a power of attorney can be formulated only while the "principal" still has the capacity to make decisions and is revoked as soon the "principal" loses their capacity. For the purposes of advance directives and future healthcare decision-making, a special provision was made wherein the power of attorney would continue to hold even after the principal lost their decision-making capacity, referred to as a "Durable Power of Attorney" (DPoA) [16].

The DPoA is a document in which the "principal" appoints another trusted person to make healthcare decisions on their behalf, if they are rendered incapacitated in future. A DPoA can be appointed only while the "principal" still has the capacity and is generally the spouse, next of kin, or a close friend. The decisional powers vested in the DPoA can be very limited or broad depending on what has been specified by the "principal." If the "principal" wants the "agent" to give their own input into making the decision, the "principal" can allow the "agent" a certain degree of leeway in the decision-making process. A DPoA has an advantage of decisions being made in keeping with the current circumstances as opposed to the hypothetical scenarios, as in the Living Will. A DPoA can also be revoked or changed as long as person still has decision-making capacity (Table 8.2).

TABLE 8.2 Termination of power of attorney [19]

If the principal dies
If the principal becomes incapacitated and the POA is not durable
If the principal revokes the POA
If the POA provides that it terminates on a specified date
If the purpose of the POA is accomplished
If the agent dies, becomes incapacitated, or resigns and the POA does not provide for another agent to act under the POA

Physician Orders for Life-Sustaining Treatment

Advance directives, even when in place, are not always followed when needed if there is no clear indication of the document's availability. Physician Orders for Life-Sustaining Treatment (POLST) was started in Oregon in 1991 to help ensure implementation of patient's end-of-life preferences [18]. It is mostly used when a patient is diagnosed with a terminal disease. POLST is a medical form wherein the doctor "prescribes" patient's preferred care and end-of-life treatment options. It starts with a conversation between a patient and the doctor about the patient's end-of-life treatment choices, which are then written on a standardized POLST form and signed by the doctor. The POLST is followed like a doctor's orders [20]. This form stays and travels with the patient as a part of their medical record. The POLST paradigm recognizes that allowing natural death to occur is not the same as killing, and it does not allow for active euthanasia or clinician-assisted suicide.

POLST is now a national movement, implemented at the state level, that supports patient autonomy regarding treatment preferences during a medical emergency. As of 2017, the National POLST Paradigm Program had been adopted by 24 states and 21 other states were in the process of developing this program [21]. Evidence suggests that while the use of this form has been helpful in successfully following patient's preferences for cardiopulmonary resuscitation, there continues to be discordance in care provided vis-a-vis level of medical intervention, antibiotics, and artificial nutrition [22].

Factors Affecting the Completion of Advance Directives

In a systematic review of the studies published between 2011 and 2016 to determine the proportion of US adults [22, 23] with completed advance directives (ADs), only 1 in 3 older adults were found to have completed some form of ADs [24]. Of the of 795,909 people analyzed, 36.7% had completed an advance directive, including 29.3% with living wills. Similar proportions of patients with chronic illnesses (38.2%) and healthy adults (32.7%) had completed advance directives. The study also found that the completion was highest among patients who were ≥65 years of age (45.6%) and patients who were in hospice or palliative care (59.6%) and in nursing homes (50.1%). Patients with neurological illnesses had highest rates of completions of ADs compared to lowest among people with HIV/AIDS. Existing literature shows a consistent trend of higher advance directives completion rate among non-Hispanic Whites when compared to African Americans, the reasons for which are not entirely clear [12, 24, 25]. One study suggests the role of cultural values in completing advance directives among Latinos and Asian Americans, while spirituality and religion are found to play a more important role among African Americans [26] (Table 8.3).

Conversations between healthcare providers, patients, and families are found to be key in improving AD completion rates [6]. Placing less emphasis on completing paperwork and completing legal formalities and being able to communicate choices orally to the clinician reduces the burden on patients and families and hence improve the planning process.

TABLE 8.3 Factors affecting completion of advance directives

Patient and family related	Clinician related
Ignorance about availability of ADs [27]	Lack of training in communicating end of life issues [28]
Reluctance and hesitation to talk about death [28]	Insufficient time [29]
Difficulty completing paperwork [27]	Difficulty estimating prognosis and timing these conversations [28]
Discordance in treatment preferences with surrogates/ family members [27]	Communication barriers and cultural differences [28]
Legal/document related	Healthcare system related
Difficulty understanding laws and language in the document [28]	Lack of a designated person responsible for initiating these conversations [28]
	Availability of ADs when needed due to different venues providing care [28]

Clinician training and education, addressing barriers in completion of ADs with families, writing ADs in simple language that is easily comprehensible are other solutions that may help AD completion rates.

Benefits of Advance Healthcare Planning

Advance healthcare planning has been shown to be beneficial for patients and caregivers while reducing the burden on healthcare system, the legal system, and the economy. As opposed to a long-standing fear of delivering bad news and causing psychological distress to the patients and their families from having end-of-life care discussion [30], recent studies show a better quality of life at the end of life among individuals engaged in these discussions early on in their care [31]. A longitudinal study with terminal cancer patients showed that patients who reported end-of-life conversations were significantly more likely to accept that their illness was terminal, prefer palliative over life-prolonging measures, and complete a do-not-resuscitate order. They also received significantly fewer aggressive medical interventions near death. Additionally, patients reporting end-of-life discussions were more likely to be enrolled in outpatient hospice care for more than 1 week where patient's quality of life improved the longer they were enrolled, except for patients who received less than 1 week of services.

Patients with cancer who die in a hospital or in an intensive care unit (ICU) have worse quality of life when compared with those who die at home, and their bereaved caregivers are at increased risk for developing psychiatric illness [32]. Caregivers of patients who had advance directives in place also reported reduced stress and anxiety at the time of death of their loved one [33]. Caregivers of patients who received any aggressive care were at higher risk for developing a major depressive disorder, experiencing regret, and feeling unprepared for the patient's death when compared to caregivers of patients who did not receive aggressive care. Advance directives not only decrease the decision-making burden on caregivers and clinicians but also reduce the legal burden of appointing conservators. From an economic perspective, advance directives reduce the cost of care by reducing unnecessary costly procedures. Six such studies found reductions in costs of care ranging from USD1041 to USD64,827 per patient, depending on the study period and the cost measurement, whereas only one study detected no differences in costs [32].

Limitations of Advance Healthcare Planning

Despite the appeal of advance healthcare planning and enthusiasm in promoting them, it suffers from important practical limitations [34]. A fundamental issue with advance healthcare planning is poor predictability in one's own future care decisions. People may formulate their ADs with hypothetical scenarios in mind, but real-life situations may be very different from what they had imagined, under which they may have made completely different treatment choices.

Furthermore, not everyone formulating their advance directives may be consistent in their end-of-life treatment preferences and patients may change their mind about their care choices with changes in health status [35]. A systematic review found that end-of-care preference stability was generally greater among inpatients and seriously ill outpatients than among older adults without serious illnesses [36]. Multiple different factors including demographic, psychological, and those pertaining to disease course have been noted to influence the stability of treatment choices. Unfortunately, changes in treatment preferences over time, especially if not communicated appropriately, may violate the very autonomy that advance care planning was designed to protect, thus threatening its utility.

Similar inaccuracies have also been noted in decisions made by surrogates on patient's behalf when chosen as their power of attorney. A meta-analysis demonstrated that surrogates predicted patients' treatment preferences with only 68% accuracy, and neither patient designation of surrogates nor prior discussion of patients' treatment preferences improved surrogates' predictive accuracy [37].

Another criticism of advance directives is often the way they are written. Some advance directives default to aggressive life-saving measures and patients are required to opt in for more palliative measures, which could influence the patient's choices [35]. Many advance directives are ambivalent such that it may be difficult to interpret or execute those under a specific clinical scenario. Sometimes the language is confusing such that it may be clear to the clinician who helped formulate the advance directives, but it may not be comprehensible to the healthcare providers who are responsible for implementing the advance directives if the patient is in a different healthcare setting at the end of life [34].

Finally, research indicates discordance in advance care preferences stated by the patient and the care received by them at the end of life [38]. A common reason for this discordance is the unavailability of advance directives in patient's medical records. Patients often receive end-of-life care in a venue different than where they formulated their advance directives and the healthcare team providing care at end of life may have no knowledge of its existence. Even when healthcare providers know about advance directives for a patient, they are sometimes not followed due to several clinician-related reasons. Clinicians may sometimes assume that they know what the patient would have wanted, rather than looking at the ADs. Furthermore, even if they know the patient did not want life-sustaining measures, they may hesitate to withdraw these measures due to their personal preferences and attitude, especially if the family members question the withdrawal or due to fear of litigation [39]. It is important for clinicians to bear in mind that advance directives are legally binding and that patients and families can sue them if they are not followed, as seen in the case of *Estate of Leach* vs. *Shapiro* (1984). It is advisable to involve hospital ethical committees and courts in matters of ambiguous advance directives, rather than defaulting to life-sustaining measures.

Novel Approaches

Due to the above-mentioned shortcomings of current advance healthcare planning, research is underway to find ways to increase AD completion rates, to uphold its goals, and effect their implementation [40, 41]. Some newer models have been implemented to overcome the limitations of the current planning process. The best-known model is the "Five Wishes," which addresses a person's personal, emotional, spiritual, and medical wishes and is more versatile and comprehensive than the traditional Living Will documents. It currently meets the statutory criteria in 42 US states. Another program called "Respecting Choices" was started in Wisconsin, USA, in 1991 as a part of community-wide care planning system. Under this program, healthcare professionals received trainings to improve communication about care planning, quality improvement projects were undertaken to improve outcomes, and efforts were made by local healthcare institutes to have advance directives available in patient's medical records at all times. A systematic review shows there is a high level of evidence that "Respecting Choices" and similar models increase patient-surrogate congruence in Caucasian populations. However, the evidence is mixed, inconclusive, and too poor in quality to determine whether they change the consistency of treatment with wishes and the overall healthcare utilization at the end of life [42].

Online Resources for Clinicians and Patients

1. Advance healthcare planning guide: https://www.nia.nih.gov/health/advance-care-planning-healthcare-directives
2. POLST educational videos: https://polst.org/polst-education-videos/
3. Advance directive forms by state: http://www.caringinfo.org/i4a/pages/index.cfm?pageid=3289
4. Information on Advance Directives registries: https://www.americanbar.org/groups/law_aging/publications/bifocal/vol_37/issue_6_august2016/tour-of-state-advance-directive-registries/
5. Patient-centered advance care planning tool guides [5, 43]:

   (a) Advance care planning toolkit by American Bar Association: https://www.americanbar.org/groups/law_aging/resources/health_care_decision_making/consumer_s_toolkit_for_health_care_advance_planning/
   (b) Making Your Wishes Known, an online tool for advance care planning: https://www.makingyourwishesknown.com
   (c) PREPARE, a web site with videos to help prepare patients for decision-making: https://www.prepareforyourcare.org/welcome
   (d) ACP Decisions, videos for patients and surrogates about goals of care, and end-of-life treatment options: https://acpdecisions.org
   (e) The Conversation Project: http://theconversationproject.org
   (f) The *GO WISH* Card Game: http://www.gowish.org

Conclusions

Advance healthcare planning has become essential and relevant in the care of older adults given their complex healthcare needs. Advance healthcare planning promotes an individual's values and autonomy, while decreasing the decision-making burden on surrogates and healthcare providers. However, the process of advance healthcare planning suffers from important limitations that reduces its utility, and this issue needs to be addressed promptly. Advance healthcare planning is a shared responsibility of law and policymakers, patients, families, and the healthcare providers. These disciplines need to come together to resolve issues with advance healthcare planning, so as to maintain an individual's values and autonomy. High-quality research is needed in this field to guide next steps and improve the process of advance healthcare planning.

References

1. Multiple Chronic Conditions Chartbook [Internet]. AHRQ Publications No, Q14–0038. [cited Dec 15, 2018].
2. Crimmins EM, Beltran-Sanchez H. Mortality and morbidity trends: is there compression of morbidity? J Gerontol B Psychol Sci Soc Sci. 2011;66(1):75–86.
3. Singer PA, Robertson G, Roy DJ. Bioethics for clinicians: 6. Advance care planning. CMAJ: Can Med Assoc J= journal de l'Association medicale canadienne. 1996;155(12):1689–92.
4. Miller B. Nurses in the know: the history and future of advance directives. Online J Issues Nurs. 2017;22:3.
5. Sabatino CP. The evolution of health care advance planning law and policy. Milbank Q. 2010;88(2):211–39.
6. Sabatino CP. Advance directives and advance care planning: legal and policy issues: Office of the Assitant Secretary for Planning and Evaluation. 2007. Available from: https://aspe.hhs.gov/basic-report/advance-directives-and-advance-care-planning-legal-and-policy-issues.
7. Obade CC. Cruzan and its sequelae: the supreme court decides its first "right-to-die" case. J Clin Ethics. 1990;1(3):242–4.

8. Patient Self Determination Act of 1990, 101st Congress Sess. 1990.
9. Kelley K. The patient self-determination act. A matter of life and death. Physician Assist (American Academy of Physician Assistants). 1995;19(3):49. 53-6, 9-60 passim.
10. Centers for Medicare and Medicaid Services. Advance care planning June 2018 [cited 2018 Dec 16]. Medicare Fee-For-Service Providers]. Available from: https://www.cms.gov/Outreach-and-Education/Medicare-Learning-Network-MLN/MLNProducts/Downloads/AdvanceCarePlanning.pdf.
11. Lum HD, Sudore RL, Bekelman DB. Advance care planning in the elderly. Med Clin North Am. 2015;99(2):391–403.
12. LoPresti MA, Dement F, Gold HT. End-of-life care for people with cancer from ethnic minority groups: a systematic review. Am J Hosp Palliat Care. 2016;33(3):291–305.
13. Fahner JC, Beunders AJM, van der Heide A, Rietjens JAC, Vanderschuren MM, van Delden JJM, et al. Interventions guiding advance care planning conversations: a systematic review. J Am Med Dir Assoc. 2018;20(3):227–48.
14. Oczkowski SJ, Chung HO, Hanvey L, Mbuagbaw L, You JJ. Communication tools for end-of-life decision-making in ambulatory care settings: a systematic review and meta-analysis. PLoS One. 2016;11(4):e0150671.
15. Doukas DJ, Antonucci T, Gorenflo DW. A multigenerational study on the correlation of values and advance directives. Ethics Behav. 1992;2(1):51–9.
16. Garraty CM. Durable power of attorney for health care: a better choice. Conn Prob LJ. 1992;7(1):115–41.
17. Sabatino CP. Ten legal myths about advance medical directives. Clear Rev. 1994;28(6):653–6.
18. Schmidt TA, Olszewski EA, Zive D, Fromme EK, Tolle SW. The Oregon physician orders for life-sustaining treatment registry: a preliminary study of emergency medical services utilization. J Emerg Med. 2013;44(4):796–805.
19. South Carolina Uniform Power of Attorney Act, Termination of power of attorney or agent's authority. Jan 1, 2017.
20. Hickman SE, Keevern E, Hammes BJ. Use of the physician orders for life-sustaining treatment program in the clinical setting: a systematic review of the literature. J Am Geriatr Soc. 2015;63(2):341–50.
21. National POLST Paradigm. National POLST Paradigm. [cited 2018 Dec 23]. Available from: https://polst.org/programs-in-your-state/.

22. Hickman SE, Hammes BJ, Torke AM, Sudore RL, Sachs GA. The quality of physician orders for life-sustaining treatment decisions: a pilot study. J Palliat Med. 2017;20(2):155–62.
23. Yadav KN, Gabler NB, Cooney E, Kent S, Kim J, Herbst N, et al. Approximately one in three US adults completes any type of advance directive for end-of-life care. Health Aff (Project Hope). 2017;36(7):1244–51.
24. Koss CS, Baker TA. Race differences in advance directive completion. J Aging Health. 2017;29(2):324–42.
25. Portanova J, Ailshire J, Perez C, Rahman A, Enguidanos S. Ethnic differences in advance directive completion and care preferences: what has changed in a decade? J Am Geriatr Soc. 2017;65(6):1352–7.
26. Hong M, Yi EH, Johnson KJ, Adamek ME. Facilitators and barriers for advance care planning among ethnic and racial minorities in the U.S.: a systematic review of the current literature. J Immigr Minor Health. 2018;20(5):1277–87.
27. Glick KL, Mackay KM, Balasingam S, Dolan KR, Casper-Isaac S. Advance directives: barriers to completion. J N Y State Nurses Assoc. 1998;29(1):4–8.
28. Office of the Assistant Secretary for Planning and Evaluation. Advance directives and advance care planning: report to Congress. U.S. Department of Health and Human Services. 2008.
29. Howard M, Bernard C, Klein D, Elston D, Tan A, Slaven M, et al. Barriers to and enablers of advance care planning with patients in primary care: survey of health care providers. Can Fam Physician. 2018;64(4):e190–e8.
30. Cherlin E, Fried T, Prigerson HG, Schulman-Green D, Johnson-Hurzeler R, Bradley EH. Communication between physicians and family caregivers about care at the end of life: when do discussions occur and what is said? J Palliat Med. 2005;8(6):1176–85.
31. Wright AA, Zhang B, Ray A, Mack JW, Trice E, Balboni T, et al. Associations between end-of-life discussions, patient mental health, medical care near death, and caregiver bereavement adjustment. JAMA. 2008;300(14):1665–73.
32. Wright AA, Keating NL, Balboni TA, Matulonis UA, Block SD, Prigerson HG. Place of death: correlations with quality of life of patients with cancer and predictors of bereaved caregivers' mental health. J Clin Oncol. 2010;28(29):4457–64.
33. Detering KM, Hancock AD, Reade MC, Silvester W. The impact of advance care planning on end of life care in elderly patients: randomised controlled trial. BMJ (Clinical research ed). 2010;340:c1345.

34. Levi BH, Green MJ. Too soon to give up: re-examining the value of advance directives. Am J Bioeth: AJOB. 2010;10(4):3–22.
35. Halpern SD, Loewenstein G, Volpp KG, Cooney E, Vranas K, Quill CM, et al. Default options in advance directives influence how patients set goals for end-of-life care. Health Aff (Project Hope). 2013;32(2):408–17.
36. Auriemma CL, Nguyen CA, Bronheim R, Kent S, Nadiger S, Pardo D, et al. Stability of end-of-life preferences: a systematic review of the evidence. JAMA Intern Med. 2014;174(7):1085–92.
37. Shalowitz DI, Garrett-Mayer E, Wendler D. The accuracy of surrogate decision makers: a systematic review. Arch Intern Med. 2006;166(5):493–7.
38. Marchand L, Fowler KJ, Kokanovic O. Building successful coalitions for promoting advance care planning. Am J Hosp Palliat Care. 2006;23(2):119–26.
39. Lens V, Pollack D. Advance directives: legal remedies and psychosocial interventions. Death Stud. 2000;24(5):377–99.
40. Ramsaroop SD, Reid MC, Adelman RD. Completing an advance directive in the primary care setting: what do we need for success? J Am Geriatr Soc. 2007;55(2):277–83.
41. Josephs M, Bayard D, Gabler NB, Cooney E, Halpern SD. Active choice intervention increases advance directive completion: a randomized trial. MDM Policy Pract. 2018;3(1):2381468317753127.
42. MacKenzie MA, Smith-Howell E, Bomba PA, Meghani SH. Respecting choices and related models of advance care planning: a systematic review of published evidence. Am J Hosp Palliat Care. 2018;35(6):897–907.
43. Lum HD, Sudore RL. Advance care planning and goals of care communication in older adults with cardiovascular disease and multi-morbidity. Clin Geriatr Med. 2016;32(2):247–60.

Chapter 9
Surrogate Decision-Making

Romika Dhar and Aarti Gupta

Introduction

Current demographic trends are indicative of an aging population with the number of seniors in the United States expected to double in the next four decades [1]. The remarkable advancements in modern medicine have led to increased life expectancy on the one hand but potential for increased disease burden on the other. It is vital that as people age, individuals, families, and physicians engage in meaningful communication regarding an individual's health care and end-of-life care wishes. However, the current statistics are

R. Dhar (✉)
Department of Medicine, West Virginia University School of Medicine, Morgantown, WV, USA
e-mail: romika.dhar@hsc.wvu.edu

A. Gupta
Yale University School of Medicine, New Haven, CT, USA

© Springer Nature Switzerland AG 2019   141
M. Balasubramaniam et al. (eds.), *Psychiatric Ethics in Late-Life Patients*, https://doi.org/10.1007/978-3-030-15172-0_9

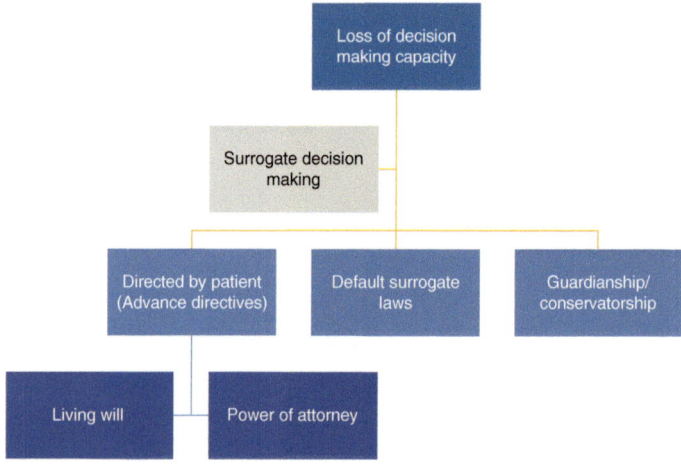

FIGURE 9.1 Different ways to appoint a surrogate decision-maker in absence of decision-making capacity

unpromising, two out of three US adults have not completed any advanced directive [2].

In the last few decades, the ethical standards for medical care have seen a paradigm shift from paternalism toward maintaining and protecting patient autonomy. Individuals can make decisions preemptively or choose a surrogate while they still have capacity through the process of advance health care planning and advance directives. In the absence of advance care directives, most individuals inadvertently rely on their state's default surrogate consent statutes. These statutes grant a person or particular class of people, usually in kinship priority, the default authority to make health care decisions for a loved one when that loved one loses decisional capacity (see Fig. 9.1).

Advance Directives

As detailed in the chapter "Advance Health Care Planning," individuals may make their own decisions preemptively and choose their own surrogate while they still have decisional capacity. This is the best way of preserving autonomy, although this is limited by its own shortcomings. If no advance directives are in place, then the default surrogate laws are applicable.

Default Surrogate Statutes

Hierarchy Surrogate Consent Laws

Majority of states have adopted the hierarchical scheme for health care surrogate appointment if the individual loses capacity and does not have advance directives. Members of the individual's family fall within a priority list of potential surrogates who may act as surrogates. In most states, the following persons are designated to serve as surrogates. In descending order of hierarch, they are the spouse (unless divorced or legally separated); an adult child; a parent; and an adult sibling. Many states include adult grand-children [3], adult nieces and nephews [4], adult uncles and aunts [5], grandparents [6], and cousins [7].

Resolving Conflict Among Surrogates

Most states provide opportunities for resolution of differences when equal priority surrogates are unable to reach a consensus regarding health care decisions or when some interested party objects to the process or decision. The designation of a hierarchy is the primary strategy states use to avoid disputes, because those lower in the hierarchy cannot overrule the authorized surrogate without resorting to judicial proceedings.

The most common provision for dispute resolution among multiple surrogates at the same level of authority (typically adult children) is to allow clinicians to rely on a majority of the equally authorized surrogates. A second model for dispute resolution contained in two states' statutes (Delaware and Maryland) is the referral to and reliance on the recommendation of an ethics committee. Although ethics committees can play a valuable role in improving policy and practice, committees are seldom quick or qualified enough to play a meaningful role in real-time, bedside decisions [8, 9]. In West Virginia and Tennessee, the health care provider can select a surrogate who appears to be best qualified based on reasonable inquiry [10, 11].

Even without an express provision for resolving disagreements, judicial intervention through the initiation of a guardianship or conservatorship is always available as a possible intervention by any interested party.

Pitfalls in Hierarchy Surrogate Consent Laws

Health care team may not look to a lower-ordered potential surrogate (e.g., sibling) if a higher-ordered potential surrogate (e.g., spouse) is available, capable, and is willing to serve as a surrogate. However, this order does not correlate with who will be the best qualified surrogate. Even in traditional family structures, the legal hierarchy may not reflect reality where families are geographically apart or complicated by divorce and remarriage, or where a friend has become the closest confidante and supporter. This supports the concept of the best qualified surrogate, who might be at the bottom of the hierarchical list, but the one that the health care team identifies as an "adult who has exhibited special care and concern for the individual, who is familiar with the individual's personal values, who is reasonably available, and who is willing to serve."

Some states have taken into account such factors in formulating laws regarding surrogate appointments. In Tennessee [12], the hierarchical list is simply something to which "consideration may be given in order of descending preference for service as a surrogate." The Tennessee statute provides five mandatory criteria for determination of the person best qualified to serve as the surrogate: (1) whether the proposed surrogate reasonably appears to be better able to make decisions either in accordance with the known wishes of the individual or in accordance with the patient's best interests; (2) the proposed surrogate's regular contact with the individual prior to and during the incapacitating illness; (3) the proposed surrogate's demonstrated care and concern; (4) the proposed surrogate's availability to visit the individual during the individual's illness; and (5) the proposed surrogate's availability to engage in face-to-face contact with health care providers for the purpose of fully participating in the decision-making process.

Colorado and Hawaii have chosen an alternative to reliance on a hierarchy list by creating a single class of "interested persons" [13, 14]. In Hawaii, "interested persons" includes the individual's spouse (unless legally separated or estranged), a reciprocal beneficiary, any adult child, either parent of the individual, an adult sibling or adult grandchild of the individual, or any adult who has exhibited special care and concern for the individual and who is familiar with the individual's personal values.

At the time of writing this chapter, Missouri, Rhode Island, and Massachusetts do not have a default hierarchical list for the selection of surrogates. Any available next of kin is appointed as a surrogate, and if there is a dispute, judicial intervention is sought. In California, Kansas, New Jersey, and Oklahoma, the laws only apply for consenting to medical research. The surrogate consent statute in Wisconsin only applies to certain facility admissions.

Status and Recognition of Domestic Partner as Default Surrogate in Non-traditional Families

The surrogates list in a majority of the states fails to include domestic partners who are not legally married. While a same-sex partner would probably qualify as a "close friend" in some of these states, that category is usually listed only at the bottom of the surrogate list [15].

Only 15 states have an LGBTQ-inclusive surrogate selection statute. Because an individual's same-sex or domestic partner often has greater knowledge of the individual's values than statutorily recognized decision-makers, such as estranged family, disregarding the partner's input is considered to be unethical [16].

Status of the Unbefriended

Fourteen states have enacted provisions for decisionally incapable individuals who have no living relative or friend who can be involved in the decision-making. This class of individuals is referred to as the "unbefriended" [17].

The unbefriended individual includes "persons who are decisionally incapacitated" and is made up of two main groups:

1. Those who had capacity and lost it, including frail elders in nursing homes and hospitals
2. Those who never had capacity, including persons with mental retardation or developmental disabilities.

In nine states, attending and primary physicians have been placed on surrogate priority lists for patients with no family or friend surrogates. These states typically seek to prevent unilateral decision-making by requiring physicians to consult an ethics committee or have the concurrence of a second physician before health care decisions are made for the unbefriended.

Given the vulnerable nature of this population, clinicians, health care teams, and ethicists must be diligent when formulating treatment decisions on their behalf. Public guardianship is often one of the avenues that is resorted to for this population. In the majority of US states, public guardianship programs are managed through a social service agency or county government public officials. However, this is less than ideal solution as it is unclear what caliber of decision-making guardians can provide. Another variation is the ability to apply for temporary and emergency guardianships when there is no time to conduct normal "plenary" or full guardianship hearings, which may take several weeks or months [18].

The American Geriatrics society has published a position statement on making medical treatment decisions for unbefriended older adults [19]. The statement proposes that the process of arriving at a treatment decision for an unbefriended older adult should be conducted according to the standards of procedural fairness and include capacity assessment, a search for potentially unidentified surrogate decision-makers, and a team-based effort to ascertain the unbefriended older adult's preferences by synthesizing all available evidence. Proactive preventive efforts are also needed to reduce older adults' risk of becoming unbefriended.

Guardianship

If no advance directives or qualified surrogates are available, or in the absence of default surrogate laws, a guardian is appointed through a legal due process. This step is used as one of last resort due to the vast delegation of powers to the guardian. Please refer to the chapter on Guardianship for more details.

Standards for Surrogate Decision-Making

Substituted Judgment Standard

In a majority of states, surrogates must make decisions in accordance with a substituted judgment standard [20]. Per this standard, the surrogates try to make the decision that the individual would have made if he or she were able to make decisions even if such wishes may not have been expressly conveyed.

The appeal of this standard is that it supports the individual's autonomy by leading us to the decision that the individual would have wanted. However, several authors have argued that substituted judgment does not succeed in meeting this goal due to several reasons [21–23].

Individuals' own preferences regarding life-sustaining treatment change over time. In one study, over half of individuals who initially said yes to a series of medical procedures changed their minds over the next 2 years [24]. However, individuals who had made advanced directives were less likely to change their wishes than those who do not [25]. Thus, the individuals who most need substituted judgment, because they lack a living will, are the ones for whom it is least likely to be accurate.

A meta-analysis of surrogate predictions found that that surrogates make different decisions than individuals would make for themselves in roughly one-third of cases [26]. Research also suggests that surrogates' own treatment preferences may influence their predictions of others' preferences. Evidence also indicates that surrogate predictions more closely resemble surrogates' own treatment wishes rather than the wishes of the individual that they were trying to predict [27]. Intense emotional distress and impaired information processing have been implicated in reducing a surrogate decision-maker's ability to formulate informed health care decisions for a critically ill patient [28].

The Best Interest Standard

The best interest standard seeks to implement one's best interests by reflecting upon the welfare or wellbeing of the individual [29]. If the individual's wishes cannot be ascertained or inferred in any way, the surrogate is obligated to make a decision consistent with what *most* people would decide for themselves under the same circumstances, or what would be best for the individual.

Dignity-driven decision-making is an important emerging concept based on respect for persons defined as "a process in which decisions about the patient's care emerge from a collaborative relationship developed over multiple encounters." This method favors patient autonomy and greater support for surrogate decision-makers [30]. Care that features dignity-driven decision-making involves balancing medical care with supportive services.

A shared decision-making model implemented early in treatment with surrogates and health care providers working together to effectively prepare for and tackle the multiple issues surrounding benefits and burdens of treatment to the individual is very important.

Special Considerations in Surrogate Decision-Making

To protect against the potential abuse of incapacitated adults, some states have placed limitations on surrogate decision-making. The District of Columbia has adopted a procedural limitation requiring that at least one witness be present whenever a surrogate grants, refuses, or withdraws consent on behalf of the individual [31].

About a dozen states permit surrogates to withhold life-sustaining treatment only if the individual has been certified to be in a terminal or permanently unconscious condition [32]. Many states impose stricter conditions to the withholding of artificial nutrition and hydration. Ohio prohibits withholding artificial nutrition and hydration unless there is a mandated court order [33].

Health care decisions statutes often treat artificial nutrition and hydration differently from other forms of life-sustaining medical treatment. Many states impose special additional conditions on surrogate decisions to withhold or withdraw artificial nutrition and hydration [34].

Conclusions

Surrogate decision-making is a crucial tool for delivering medical care to older adults lacking decisional capacity. In the absence of advance health care directives, default surrogate laws or guardianship are resorted to maintain the safety of the older adult. Default surrogate statutes of hierarchical order of surrogate selection are a helpful concept in the time of need, but have some practical limitations that need to be addressed. There is need for flexibility in prioritizing interested persons who are familiar with the individual's personal values and care goals as opposed to choosing surrogates based on blood or marital relationships. Furthermore, these laws may need to be revamped to accommodate the increasingly common non-traditional family structures.

Surrogate decision-making, although currently widely utilized, is criticized for its inability to make accurate decisions for an incapacitated person. Though different models have been proposed over the years to circumvent the shortcomings of surrogate decision-making, some of the pitfalls are unavoidable. Shared decision-making, a collaborative process that allows individuals, their surrogates, and clinicians to make health care decisions together, taking into account the best scientific evidence available, as well as the individuals' values, goals, and preferences if known, may help in dealing with this challenging problem. The next step is high-quality research trials studying the feasibility and impact of this intervention on older individuals, their families, and the health care system.

References

1. https://www.census.gov/prod/2010pubs/p25-1138.pdf. Accessed 17 Nov 2018.
2. Yadav KN, Gabler NB. Approximately one in three US adults completes any type of advance directive for end-of-life care. Health Aff. 2017;36(7):1244.
3. Del. Code. Ann., tit. 16 § 2507(b)(2)(e); Ga. Code Ann. § 31-9-2(a) (6)(E); 755 Ill. Comp. Stat. 40/25(a)(6); Me. Rev. Stat., tit. 18A§ 5-805(b)(5); Pa. Stat. Ann., tit. 20 § 5461(d)(1)(v); S.C. Code Ann. § 44-66-30(A)(6); S.D. Codified Laws § 34-12C-3(5); Utah Code Ann.§ 75-2a-108(1)(b)(ii)(D);Wis. Stat. Ann. § 50.06(3)(f); Wyo. Stat. §35-22-406(b)(vi).
4. Del. Code. Ann., tit. 16 § 2507(b)(2)(f); Ga. Code Ann. § 31-9-2(a) (6)(F); Me. Rev. Stat., tit. 18A § 5-805(b)(6); S.D. Codified Laws § 34-12C-3(6).
5. Ga. Code Ann. § 31-9-2(a)(6)(F); Me. Rev. Stat., tit. 18A §5-805(b) (7); S.D. Codified Laws § 34-12C-3(6).

6. Ga. Code Ann. § 31-9-2(a)(6)(D); N.M. Stat. Ann. §24-7A-5(B) (6); S.C. Code Ann. § 44-66-30(A)(6); S.D. Codified Laws § 34-12C-3(5); Utah Code Ann. § 75-2a-108(1)(b)(ii)(F); Wis.Stat. Ann. § 50.06(3)(e); Wyo. Stat. § 35-22-406(b)(iv).
7. S.D. Codified Laws § 34-12C-3(6).
8. Del. Code § 2507(b)(9).
9. Maryland Code, Health-Gen. § 5-605(b).
10. Tenn. Code Ann. § 68-11-1806(c).
11. W. Va. Code, § 16-30-8(b).
12. Tenn. Code Ann. § 68-11-1806(c)(3).
13. Hawaii Rev. Stat. §572-C-.
14. Colo. Rev. Stat. Ann. § 15-18.5-103(3).
15. Alaska Stat. § 47.24.016(a)(6); Ark. Rev. Stat. § 36-3231(A)(6); Del. Code Ann., tit. 16 § 2507(b)(3); Fla. Stat. Ann. § 765.401(1) (g); W. Va. Code § 16-30-8(a)(6).
16. Castillo LS, Williams BA, Hooper SM, Sabatino CP, Weithorn LA, Sudore RL. Lost in translation: the unintended consequences of advance directive law on clinical care. Ann Intern Med. 2011;154(2):121–8.
17. Karp N, Wood E. Incapacitated and alone: medical decision-making for the unbefriended elderly. Washington, DC: American Bar Association Commission on Law and Aging; 2003.
18. Cal. prob. code § 3208 (west 2016); Fla. prob. rule 5.900 (2017); O.C.G.A § 31-36a-7 (2016) (placement only); Ind. code § 16-36-1-8 (2016); N.J ct. rule 4:86-12 (2016) (special medical guardian); S.D. codified laws. § 34-12c-4 (2016); VA code ann. § 37.2-1101(b) (west2016), amended by s.b. 371, 2012 gen. assemb., reg. sess. (va. 2012).
19. Farrell TW, Widera E, Rosenberg L, Rubin CD, Naik AD, Braun U, et al. AGS position statement: making medical treatment decisions for unbefriended older adults. J Am Geriatr Soc. 2017;65:14–5.
20. Meisel A, Cerminara KL. The right to die: the law of end-of-life decision making. 3rd ed. New York: Aspen Publishers; 2004. p. 4.02(B)–3(B).
21. Bailey S. Decision making in health care: limitations of the substituted judgment principle. Nurs Ethics. 2002;9(5):483–9.
22. Dresser R. Precommitment: a misguided strategy for securing death with dignity. Tex Law Rev. 2003;81(7):1823–47.
23. Welie JV. Living wills and substituted judgments: a critical analysis. Med Health Care Philos. 2001;4(2):169–83.
24. Danis M, Garrett J, Harris R, Patrick DL. Stability of choices about life-sustaining treatments. Ann Intern Med. 1994;120(7):567–73.

25. Weissman JS, Haas JS, Fowler FJ Jr, et al. The stability of preferences for life-sustaining care among persons with AIDS in the Boston Health Study. Med Decis Making. 1999;19(1):16.
26. Shalowitz DI, Garrett-Mayer E, Wendler D. The accuracy of surrogate decision makers: a systematic review. Arch Intern Med. 2006;166(5):493–7.
27. Fagerlin A, Ditto PH, Danks JH, Houts RM. Projection in surrogate decisions about life-sustaining medical treatments. Health Psychol. 2001;20(3):166–75.
28. Hickman RL Jr, Pignatiello GA, Tahir S. Evaluation of the decisional fatigue scale among surrogate decision makers of the critically ill. West J Nurs Res. 2018;40(2):191–208.
29. Kopelman LM. The best interests standard for incompetent or incapacitated persons of all ages. J Law Med Ethics. 2007;35:187–96.
30. Vladeck BC, Westphal E. Dignity-driven decision making: a compelling strategy for improving care for people with advanced illness. Health Aff. 2012;31(6):1269–76.
31. DC Code § 21-2210.
32. Ala. Code § 22-8A-11(a)(2); Del. Code. tit. 16 § 2507(b)(6); Iowa Code Ann. § 144A.7(1); Me. Rev.Stat. tit. 18-A § 5-805(a); Mont. Code Ann. § 50-9-106(1)(a); Nev.Rev. Stat. § 449.626(1)(a); N.C. Gen. Stat. § 90-322(a)(1a); Ohio Rev.Code § 2133.08(D)(2).
33. Ohio Rev. Code Ann. § 2133.09.
34. Seiger CE, Arnold JF, Ahronheim JC. Refusing artificial and hydration: does statutory law send the wrong message? J Am Geriatr Soc. 2002;50(3):544–50.

Chapter 10
Guardianship

Nery A. Diaz and Reema D. Mehta

Introduction

Guardianship is a legal process utilized when individuals can no longer make or communicate sound decisions about their person or property or have become susceptible to fraud or undue influence from others [1]. When individuals are no longer able to make decisions for themselves, a court-appointed decision-maker, referred to as a "guardian," is often

N. A. Diaz (✉)
Columbia University Irving Medical Center, New York, NY, USA

New York State Psychiatric Institute, New York, NY, USA
e-mail: nad2149@cumc.columbia.edu

R. D. Mehta
Jacobi Medical Center, Bronx, NY, USA

Albert Einstein College of Medicine, Bronx, NY, USA
e-mail: Reema.Mehta@nychhc.org

© Springer Nature Switzerland AG 2019   153
M. Balasubramaniam et al. (eds.), *Psychiatric Ethics in Late-Life Patients*, https://doi.org/10.1007/978-3-030-15172-0_10

appointed to make decisions on their behalf [2]. The person for whom the guardian is appointed is referred to as a "ward." There are different types of guardianship, including guardianship of person, guardianship of estate, or both. In many states, the term "conservator" is used interchangeably with "guardian." For ease of reference, in this chapter, the term "guardian" is used to describe a court-appointed decision-maker.

Physician's Role in Guardianship

Evaluating Decision-Making Capacity

Decision-making capacity is the key area to be assessed when evaluating an individual who appears to be in need for a guardian [3]. The assessment of decisional capacity includes an individual's ability to communicate a clear choice, understand relevant information, appreciate the situation and its consequences, and manipulate the information rationally [4]. The clinician should also assess whether these individuals are maintaining consistent decisions and their primary values over time.

Decision-making capacity is not a global construct, but something that is situation specific and time limited [4]. For example, scenarios may arise in which an individual has the capacity to make medical decisions, but not financial decisions, or vice versa. The initial step in assessing decisional capacity is to identify areas where the individual may not be able to make sound decisions for themselves, such as finance, health care, sexual relations, or independent living [5]. This evaluation is important as it will assist the courts in limiting the guardianship to only the areas in which the older adult lacks decisional capacity. Guardianship may be limited to only property, only finance, only medical decision-making, or some combination of these areas as is deemed appropriate for each individual.

When evaluating an individual's financial decision-making capacity, their ability to manage accounts, assets, and benefits must be identified and clearly documented. Clinicians are also required to comment on the vulnerability of the older adult to financial exploitation while making their assessment [6]. Although more research is needed to identify instruments that can aide in the evaluation of financial capacity, one tool available is the *Semi-Structured Clinical Interview for Financial Capacity* [7].

Often clinicians are asked to assess an individual's ability to reside independently in the community. In these cases, it is important to pay particular attention to the individuals' abilities to maintain a safe living environment, including their ability to seek help in case of an emergency. The Functional Activities Questionnaire is an efficient tool for assessing an individual's ability to function independently [8].

In addition, the clinician may want to consider an individual's ability to make safe decisions about sexual relationships [9]. The ethical and safety considerations of sexual relations involving persons with dementing illness are the subject of grave concern for their families and residential care facilities. Ethical principles support decisions made on a case-by-case basis, guided by a respect for the autonomy of the patient that is balanced with informed consent [10]. If an older adult is making decisions about sexual relationships that are inconsistent and defy their value system, however, and their capacity to make these decisions appears impaired, then the need for a guardian should be considered.

A unique area of evaluation among older adults is that of abuse, neglect, and self-neglect. Abuse and neglect of older adults occur in about 5 million older adults each year in the United States [11]. Self-neglect is a serious problem that is excluded from most state adult protective service (APS) abuse registries [12]. Self-neglect is defined as the "behavior of an elder person that threatens his/her own health or safety [13]." Among these individuals, the capacity to make personal decisions may remain intact, but their ability to remove themselves from harmful situations or persons who can cause harm may be diminished. Obtaining collateral information from a reliable third party is very important in the determination of capacity among older adults who are suspected of self-neglect [14, 15].

Capacity Restoration

If an individual lacks decision-making capacity, then it is essential to determine whether the capacity can be restored by reversing the conditions that have led to the incapacity [3]. If they are reversible, then the clinician should seek to do so and advise postponing any guardianship decisions until the precipitating conditions have improved.

The clinician should recognize that medical conditions such as infections, dehydration, delirium, poor oral care, malnutrition, and pain can be treated and improved with appropriate medical care [16, 17]. If hearing or vision loss is the underlying cause for the concerns, the clinician should make the appropriate referrals to manage these sensory deficits [18, 19]. Medication side effects can result in older adults developing temporary cognitive deficits that impair their decision-making ability [20, 21]. These temporary cognitive deficits can often be reversed when the offending agents are discontinued. Clinicians should avoid using medications on the Beers Criteria that are deemed potentially inappropriate for use among older adults [22].

Injudicious polypharmacy in the elderly population is a major area of concern and should be managed carefully [22]. Medication lists should be reviewed thoroughly to ensure that the older individual is not receiving medications that were discontinued previously or is currently receiving medications that are harmful to the individual.

Clinicians should also evaluate the individual's psychological conditions, including stressors, grief, depression, and disorientation [23, 24]. They should keep in mind that improving physical condition, enhancing self-efficacy, and increasing engagement in healthy behaviors are factors that may account for why some older persons recover from disability while others struggle to do so [25]. If the concerns regarding decisional capacity are temporary, guardians can be appointed for a specific role or for limited time. This role is often referred to as the "Special Limited Conservator." For example, a guardianship might be needed for a specific treatment that is time-limited, such as electroconvulsive therapy, or for an illness from which that person is expected to recover. However, if the underlying cause for the impairment in decisional capacity cannot be reversed, or the condition is expected to progress as is the case of a major neurocognitive disorder (dementia), then the guardianship could be indefinite.

Furthermore, the individual's decisional capacity may change with time [26]. Sometimes, the decisional capacity may improve, and other times they can become incapacitated in different ways as their health deteriorates. Therefore, clinicians should periodically reassess the decisional capacity of individuals placed under guardianships, to assess whether the individual's decisional capacity can be restored or whether further protection is necessary to prevent exploitation.

Process of Appointing a Guardian

Guardianship is frequently requested by close relatives or community providers of older individuals as they notice changes from baseline functioning and experience challenges in providing care due to an individual's lack of decision-making capacity [2, 3]. Sometimes, the need for guardianship is recognized in hospital settings, most often for treatment decision-making or discharge placement due to lack of individual's ability to provide informed consent or participate in discharge planning. In these cases, petitions are initiated by the healthcare team through the hospital's legal services. In one retrospective cohort study assessing the guardianship process for incapacitated hospitalized adults, placement was the primary reason for seeking guardianship in 88.7% of the individuals for whom guardianship was obtained [27]. In this study, the median time from a guardianship request to the appointment of a permanent guardian was 37 days, with a range of 16–71 days. In another retrospective cohort study, individuals for whom guardianship was sought had a 58% increase in length of stay and a 23% increase in hospital costs when compared to matched controls who were not awaiting guardianship [28]. In addition, 16% of the individuals awaiting appointment of a guardian had a hospital-associated complication. These studies highlight that the process of obtaining guardianship is often expensive, is time consuming, and can be deleterious to an individual's health.

Appointment of a guardian is governed by the constitutional right of an individual to due process and the guardianship statutes of each state [1]. The statutes recognize that guardianship can deprive an individual of their rights and are framed to offer protection to the proposed ward. Typically, the first step to obtaining a guardianship is filing with the court of a petition for guardianship. Due process ensures that the person who is alleged to lack decisional capacity is notified of any hearing; has the right to representation through a lawyer; is allowed to attend all hearings regarding the guardianship; can cross-examine witnesses, present, and ask for evidence supporting their lack of capacity; and sometimes has a right to a jury trial. The appointment of a guardian requires clear and convincing proof that an individual lacks decisional capacity and the absence of any less-restrictive measures short of guardianship to protect the individual's rights [1]. In some states, the court is required to review the need for continued guardianship annually and to continue to pursue less-restrictive measures to uphold the ward's rights. Wards are also allowed to request a review of their guardianship sooner, if they believe that they are no longer incapacitated.

In many cases, courts will appoint family members as guardians, either as an individual guardian or as shared decision-makers [27]. However, there may not be family members or close friends who are suitable for guardianship, perhaps due to their own medical limitations, cognitive impairment, poor relationship with the prospective ward, or unwillingness to serve as guardian for other reasons. In these cases, a judge will appoint a guardian who is unknown to the person. This guardian could be an individual or a corporation that will serve as a professional guardian [2]. Such professional guardians are often not familiar with their ward's values, preferences, and beliefs prior to them losing decision-making capacity, and they may rely on information told to them by health providers or family members. Most often, they must rely on best-interest standard in making decisions, an objective standard that does not take into account the individual's subjective wishes and values.

The guardianship process, laws, and procedures differ from state to state [29]. In addition, they have evolved over the last four decades to better protect vulnerable individuals [3]. It is, therefore, important to review local laws and procedures before petitioning the court for guardianship. Furthermore, states may differ in how they define the lack of decision-making capacity. For example, some states have general language, such as "lacks sufficient capacity to manage own affairs," while other states have additional wording, such as "even with additional support patient is unable to meet needs." To complicate matters, some states do not have any specific definitions of incapacity [29].

The American Bar Association has published a *PRACTICAL Tool for Lawyers* on guardianship [5]. This six-page pamphlet is readily available on the internet and is written in language that does not require legal training to comprehend. It is worth reviewing by any physician treating a patient facing guardianship proceedings. It is important to remember that this is a general overview and that physicians should review the statutes of their state for state-specific requirements when considering guardianship or any alternative vehicles.

Limitations to Guardian's Decision-Making

Guardianship grants a guardian broad decision-making powers over their wards [2]. To prevent indiscriminate use of this power and exploitation of the ward by the guardian, the law requires guardians to petition the courts for certain important decisions. Table 10.1 gives common examples of circumstances under which a guardian may need to obtain permission from the court, although the types of decisions requiring prior court approval can vary significantly from state to state.

In addition, state laws may differ if seeking guardianship for an adult with an intellectual or developmental disability [30]. For this reason, it is important for guardians to familiarize themselves with local laws and restrictions to decision-making [30].

TABLE 10.1 Guardian may need to petition the court for	Placing a ward in an institution
	Consenting to involuntary psychiatric medications
	Withdraw or refuse certain medical care
	Changing residence
	Changing tenancy or lease
	Sell, mortgage, or transfer real estate
	Investing funds
	Making gifts from conserved person's income or assets

Disadvantages of Guardianship

Although a guardian is appointed to safeguard the interest of an incapacitated person, there are several potential pitfalls of appointing a guardian [31]. One of the major drawbacks of guardianship is the diminution in the ward's autonomy. Even if the ward may be capable of collaborating with the guardian on certain matters, some guardians may not consult their wards before making a decision, which could undermine the ward's wishes and in turn affect their psychological wellbeing. Guardianship can also be adverse to the ward by shutting down communication between parties, shaming the ward, and potentially straining the relationship between the guardian and the ward [31].

Financial and personal abuses are another major concern due to vast delegation of powers. Popular media has uncovered several cases that highlighted significant abuse of wards' rights and financial exploitation [32]. There are also case reports in the medical literature reporting abuse and neglect at the hands of the guardian. In one such case report, a ward developed negative medical outcomes from medical neglect after the court appointed a guardian for him. The case also highlights the high monetary costs that were ordered to be paid by the wards' estate [33]. Money that is used toward guardianship costs from the ward's estate can reduce funds available to the ward for their other needs.

Even without abuse or neglect, guardianship may result in the ward's estate being managed in order to make things more convenient for the guardian and not necessarily to protect the needs of the ward [31]. Although guardians should be protecting the ward's wealth and financial wellbeing, unfortunately there is limited oversight in screening of potential guardians [34].

When the court determines the need for guardianship, the court takes these potential consequences into consideration and makes efforts to minimize potential risks to the older adult. Guardianships can be improved to better meet the needs of the individual with fewer negative consequences through the use of nonadversarial "problem-solving" courts, mediation, limiting the guardianship, building in periodic reviews, and presenting guardianship plans that outline specific goals and plans prior to the guardianship hearing [31].

Alternatives to Guardianships

As noted above, guardianship can sometimes be deleterious to the autonomy and wellbeing of the ward it is designed to protect, and it should be considered only as an intervention of last resort [31]. Accordingly, it is important for a clinician to identify less-restrictive options that can protect an individual's rights, if they are available. Although every individual's situation is unique, the following are some of the means to avoid the appointment of a guardian:

- Durable Power of Attorney for health/finance chosen per advance directives
- Healthcare surrogate under state law—the role of the surrogate is to voice the wishes of individuals who are unable to do so themselves
- Trusts
- Representative payees
- A fiduciary
- Joint bank accounts
- Case/Care management services
- Community advocacy systems
- A supporter with a representation agreement, legally or informally recognized

The clinician should discuss with the individual concerned whether other family members, professionals, or trusted friend are available to help them in any of the capacities noted above. All of these options may be superior to guardianship because the individuals themselves can dictate the terms of their life, rather than have them imposed by a court-appointed guardian.

Conclusions

When older adults lose decision-making capacity, healthcare providers should explore ways to help them regain this capacity. If the individuals' impairments in capacity cannot be restored, then alternatives to guardianship should be explored. When guardianship is necessary, then local laws and limitations should be explored before beginning the process of guardianship. While guardians are entrusted to make decisions on behalf of their ward, these decisions should be in line with the ward's wishes and values, when they are known. Although guardianship is often necessary, it is important to keep in mind the disadvantages and potential risks associated with guardianship. When guardianship is no longer necessary, the reversal of guardianship should also be explored.

References

1. National Guardianship Association. What is guardianship? Available from: https://www.guardianship.org/what-is-guardianship/.
2. Cohen AB, Wright MS, Cooney L Jr, Fried T. Guardianship and end-of-life decision making. JAMA Intern Med. 2015;175(10):1687–91.
3. Moye J, Naik AD. Preserving rights for individuals facing guardianship. JAMA. 2011;305(9):936–7.
4. Appelbaum PS, Grisso T. Assessing patients' capacities to consent to treatment. N Engl J Med. 1988;319(25):1635–8.
5. PRACTICAL Tool for Lawyers: steps in supporting decision-making. 2016. Available from: https://www.americanbar.org/content/dam/aba/administrative/law_aging/PRACTICALGuide.pdf.

6. Tueth MJ. Exposing financial exploitation of impaired elderly persons. Am J Geriatr Psychiatry. 2000;8(2):104–11.
7. Marson DC, Martin RC, Wadley V, Griffith HR, Snyder S, Goode PS, et al. Clinical interview assessment of financial capacity in older adults with mild cognitive impairment and Alzheimer's disease. J Am Geriatr Soc. 2009;57(5):806–14.
8. Pfeffer RI, Kurosaki TT, Harrah CH Jr, Chance JM, Filos S. Measurement of functional activities in older adults in the community. J Gerontol. 1982;37(3):323–9.
9. Wilkins JM. More than capacity: alternatives for sexual decision making for individuals with dementia. Gerontologist. 2015;55(5):716–23.
10. Mahieu L, Gastmans C. Sexuality in institutionalized elderly persons: a systematic review of argument-based ethics literature. Int Psychogeriatr. 2012;24(3):346–57.
11. Elder abuse facts. Available from: https://www.ncoa.org/public-policy-action/elder-justice/elder-abuse-facts/.
12. NAPSA. NAPSA Adult Protective Services Abuse Registry National Report. 2018.
13. Types of abuse [cited 2018]. Available from: https://ncea.acl.gov/faq/abusetypes.html - self.
14. Naik AD, Lai JM, Kunik ME, Dyer CB. Assessing capacity in suspected cases of self-neglect. Geriatrics. 2008;63(2):24–31.
15. Gill TM. Elder self-neglect: medical emergency or marker of extreme vulnerability? JAMA. 2009;302(5):570–1.
16. Mittal V, Muralee S, Williamson D, McEnerney N, Thomas J, Cash M, et al. Review: delirium in the elderly: a comprehensive review. Am J Alzheimers Dis Other Demen. 2011;26(2):97–109.
17. Inouye SK, Westendorp RG, Saczynski JS. Delirium in elderly people. Lancet. 2014;383(9920):911–22.
18. Yueh B, Shapiro N, MacLean CH, Shekelle PG. Screening and management of adult hearing loss in primary care: scientific review. JAMA. 2003;289(15):1976–85.
19. Rubin GS, Roche KB, Prasada-Rao P, Fried LP. Visual impairment and disability in older adults. Optom Vis Sci. 1994;71(12):750–60.
20. Ancelin ML, Artero S, Portet F, Dupuy AM, Touchon J, Ritchie K. Non-degenerative mild cognitive impairment in elderly people and use of anticholinergic drugs: longitudinal cohort study. BMJ. 2006;332(7539):455–9.
21. Mintzer J, Burns A. Anticholinergic side-effects of drugs in elderly people. J R Soc Med. 2000;93(9):457–62.
22. Fick DM, Semla TP, Beizer J, et al. American Geriatrics Society 2015 updated beers criteria for potentially inappro-

priate medication use in older adults. J Am Geriatr Soc. 2015;63(11):2227–46.

23. Kasl-Godley J, Gatz M. Psychosocial interventions for individuals with dementia: an integration of theory, therapy, and a clinical understanding of dementia. Clin Psychol Rev. 2000;20(6):755–82.

24. Block SD. Perspectives on care at the close of life. Psychological considerations, growth, and transcendence at the end of life: the art of the possible. JAMA. 2001;285(22):2898–905.

25. Levy BR, Slade MD, Murphy TE, Gill TM. Association between positive age stereotypes and recovery from disability in older persons. JAMA. 2012;308(19):1972–3.

26. Ganzini L, Volicer L, Nelson WA, Fox E, Derse AR. Ten myths about decision-making capacity. J Am Med Dir Assoc. 2005; 6(3 Suppl):S100–4.

27. Bandy RJ, Helft PR, Bandy RW, Torke AM. Medical decision-making during the guardianship process for incapacitated, hospitalized adults: a descriptive cohort study. J Gen Intern Med. 2010;25(10):1003–8.

28. Ricotta DN, Parris JJ, Parris RS, Sontag DN, Mukamal KJ. The burden of guardianship: amatched cohort study. J Hosp Med. 2018;13:595–601.

29. ABA Commission on Law and Aging. Capacity definition &initiation of guardianship proceedings American Bar Association. 2016. Available from: https://www.americanbar.org/content/dam/aba/administrative/law_aging/chartcapacityandinitiation.authcheckdam.pdf.

30. Guardianship Health Care Decision-Making Authority and Statutory Restrictions American Bar Association. 2014. Available from: https://www.americanbar.org/content/dam/aba/administrative/law_aging/2014_HealthCareDecisionMaking AuthorityofGuardiansChart.authcheckdam.pdf.

31. Wright JL. Guardianship for your own good: improving the well-being of respondents and wards in the USA. Int J Law Psychiatry. 2010;33(5–6):350–68.

32. Aviv R. How the elderly lose their rights. The New Yorker; 2017. https://www.newyorker.com/magazine/2017/10/09/how-the-elderly-lose-their-rights.

33. Edlich RF. Guardian ad litem, a potentially expensive invitation to either the mismanagement or management of patients with cognitive disorders. Clin Interv Aging. 2010;5:369–72.

34. Rabiner DJ, O'Keeffe J, Brown D. Financial exploitation of older persons: challenges and opportunities to identify, prevent, and address it in the United States. J Aging Soc Policy. 2006;18(2): 47–68.

Chapter 11
Elder Abuse

**Mary Ellen Trail Ross, Katharine L. Thomas,
Sabrina Pickens, Jennifer Bryan, and Ali Abbas Asghar-Ali**

Elder Abuse

The World Health Organization defines elder abuse as a single or repeated act, or lack of appropriate action, that causes an older person harm or distress within any relationship in

M. E. T. Ross · S. Pickens
Cizik School of Nursing, The University of Texas
Health Science Center, Houston, TX, USA
e-mail: Mary.E.Ross@uth.tmc.edu; Sabrina.L.Pickens@uth.tmc.edu

K. L. Thomas
Rice University, Houston, TX, USA
e-mail: klt2@rice.edu

J. Bryan · A. A. Asghar-Ali (✉)
VA South Central Mental Illness Research, Education and Clinical
Center, Houston, TX, USA

VA HSR&D Center for Innovations in Quality, Effectiveness and
Safety, Michael E. DeBakey VA Medical Center,
Houston, TX, USA

Department of Psychiatry, Baylor College of Medicine,
Houston, TX, USA
e-mail: Jennifer.bryan@bcm.edu; asgharal@bcm.edu

© Springer Nature Switzerland AG 2019
M. Balasubramaniam et al. (eds.), *Psychiatric Ethics in
Late-Life Patients*, https://doi.org/10.1007/978-3-030-15172-0_11

which there is an expectation of trust [30]. Elder abuse, also known as elder mistreatment, can be subdivided into five categories: physical abuse, psychological or emotional abuse, sexual abuse, financial exploitation, and neglect (caregiver and self-neglect). Nationwide, there is a 10% prevalence rate for elder abuse; however, most prevalence measurements rely heavily on self-reported data, leading researchers to believe that this number is likely underestimated [14]. It is estimated that for every case of elder abuse reported, 23 cases of elder abuse remain unreported [2]. Older adults who are more advanced in age, or mentally impaired such as suffering with dementia, socially isolated, or disabled in some way, are at a higher risk for experiencing elder abuse [21]. Addressing the gap in healthcare professionals' reporting of elder abuse is critical to the health and safety of the older adult population, as elders who experience abuse have a 300% higher risk of death [9].

As the baby-boomer generation ages and life expectancy in the United States continues to increase, the size of our elder population age 65 and older continues to rapidly expand, growing from 13.7% of the population in 2012 to an estimated 20.3% by 2020 [22]. Despite this shift to an older demographic, elder abuse research is still relatively lacking, remaining in the early stages of development. For example, despite the existence of several screening tools, identifying mistreatment is challenging because of their inconsistent use of criteria or lack of use of criteria for labeling behavior as abuse. In the remainder of the chapter, case scenarios appear in italics after the discussion for types of elder abuse.

Caregiver Neglect

The most prevalent type of elder mistreatment is neglect, with a reported one-year prevalence of 5.9% [1]. Caregiver neglect is defined as the failure of a designated caregiver to meet the needs of a dependent elder [24]. Clinically, we define a caregiver as a person in a trusting relationship with an elder who has assumed responsibility for his/her care. Abandonment, defined as "leaving an elder alone without planning for his or her care" [21] i.e. food, clothing, and shelter, is considered a form of caregiver neglect.

Mr. A, a widowed man in his late 70s, was brought into the emergency room by a neighbor who found him disoriented and wandering in the neighborhood. Upon examination, Mr. A was found to be underweight and dehydrated. He was oriented to his name only. He was unable to provide any medical history and was somewhat irritable during the interview.

The emergency room team learned that Mr. A had been diagnosed with dementia a few years earlier and that his family was responsible for his care. They were able to contact his son, who lived in a separate house in the same neighborhood as Mr. A and was the designated caregiver. Mr. A's son would come to check on Mr. A daily after he got off work and make sure that there was enough food in the house. Mr. A was home alone for most of the day. On the basis of the information provided, it appeared that Mr. A's level of care and supervision were inadequate given the extent of his cognitive deficits. The emergency room team explained to the family that Mr. A required 24-hour supervision to maintain his health and safety. They also called Adult Protective Services (APS) for concerns about neglect by Mr. A's son (as the designated caregiver).

Mr. A was admitted to treat his dehydration. During the admission, the team social worker met with Mr. A's son and worked to improve the level of care for Mr. A. The family was thankful for the education and assistance and worked with APS to secure the necessary resources to ensure that Mr. A could remain at his home with appropriate level of care.

Self-Neglect

Self-neglect is defined as the inability of an elder to perform essential self-care. Self-neglecting behavior can be due to physical or mental impairment, as well as any form of diminished capacity [16]. It can be more challenging to identify in a clinical setting because healthcare professionals are tasked with determining several factors, including whether the behavior is a recent development or part of a life-long pattern of behaviors and whether the elder has full decision-making capacity [25].

APS received a call regarding Mr. B, a 77-year-old man, who lives alone in his home. His neighbor reported concern for the state of his home, stating that there was rotten food in the fridge, no electricity, and an apparent roach infestation.

APS responded to Mr. B's home and met with Mr. B. He claimed that he was fine on his own and did not need assistance. Mr. B wanted to continue living at home. On the basis of the caseworker's clinical interview, Mr. B was oriented to self and place only. He could not explain how he procured his food, or paid his bills, or discuss any of his medical conditions or treatments. He was malodorous with soiled clothing. The house was found to be as described by the neighbor. Based on the evaluation, there was grave concern for self-neglect and Mr. B's imminent safety.

Financial Exploitation

Financial exploitation, another form of elder mistreatment, is defined as the illegal or improper use of an elder's resources for monetary or personal benefit [11]. Financial exploitation can include actions such as altering a will or life insurance policy without permission, taking someone's social security or retirement benefits, forging checks, and using someone else's credit card or bank account [21]. Financial exploitation is among the more common forms of elder mistreatment, with a one-year prevalence rate of 5.2% [1]. Financial exploitation can have severe consequences, costing adults 65 years and older approximately $36.5 billion per year and causing one in ten victims to turn to Medicaid as a result of having money stolen from them [15].

Ms. C, an 84-year-old woman, had been diagnosed with cancer earlier in the year and had asked her daughter to assist with her finances, as she no longer had the energy to take care of them. Ms. C's son visited her months later and noticed that there were a number of unpaid bills, including those for her utilities. His mother also noted that her daughter had asked her *to sign a check for $50,000 as a "loan" to the daughter. Ms. C's son became concerned about his mother's financial welfare and immediately contacted APS to report his findings.*

An investigation was opened. APS discovered that the daughter had been using her mother's accounts to pay off her own home and for other personal expenses, depleting her mother's savings. Working with Ms. C, her son, and local courts, APS was able to secure her accounts and establish her son as the responsible person for assisting his mother with her finances.

Physical Abuse

Physical abuse is defined as the willful infliction of physical force on an elder that could result in physical injury, pain, or impairment. Forms of physical abuse can include hitting, biting, kicking, pinching, forceful administration of drugs, force-feeding, physical punishment, or physical restraining of an elder [19].

Ms. D is a 72-year-old woman who recently remarried after her husband passed away several years ago. One of her sons flew into town to visit her for the weekend while her husband was away. While visiting her, Ms. D's son noticed bruising on his mother's arms and temple and thought she seemed quieter than normal. She said, "Everything is fine," when he asked her about any physical altercations or abuse.

The next day, due to his concern, Ms. D's son took her to a clinic for a physical examination by her long-standing physician. The physician found several more bruises on Ms. D's torso. With prompting, Ms. D revealed that her husband had become physically aggressive in the last six months. She had been too ashamed to share this with her physician or family. Ms. D's physician contacted APS. Ms. D was admitted to the hospital for further evaluation of her physical injuries.

Sexual Abuse

Sexual abuse is defined as nonconsensual sexual contact of any kind with an elder person, which can include acts such as unwanted touching, rape, sexually explicit photographing, and coerced nudity [19]. It is the least common form of elder mistreatment, with a one-year prevalence rate of 0.6%, although some states group sexual abuse with physical abuse, which could lead to slightly lower nationwide sexual abuse rates [1, 28]. Within group homes, perpetrators may not only be employees but also possibly other residents, often due to the prevalence of cognitive impairment disorders among those populations.

After admission, a complete physical examination was performed on Ms. D. Further evidence of abuse was discovered in the form of bruising on her inner thighs and vaginal tenderness. After the examination, Ms. D revealed that when intoxicated, her husband had been forcing her to have sex. She was not comfortable with the physician's sharing this information with her children.

The inpatient social worker and APS caseworker met with Ms. D to discuss steps to take to maintain her safety. In consultation with her children, she decided to move in with her daughter, who lived in a neighboring town.

Psychological Abuse

Psychological abuse, also known as emotional abuse, involves the infliction of anguish, pain, or distress through verbal or nonverbal acts, including insults, threats, intimidation, humiliation, harassment, or isolation [19]. It can occur in isolation or in conjunction with other forms of abuse. It is one of the more difficult forms of abuse to detect because it lacks the clear physical evidence seen with other abuse cases [10].

Mr. E is an 88-year-old man whose family recently moved him into an assisted-living facility after a fall at home, where he lived alone, several months ago. They were concerned about his safety living alone and discussed his moving into a more supported setting. Mr. E agreed and selected his new home with his family.

On a visit to their father, Mr. E's children noticed that he seemed withdrawn and was not eating as well. During the visit,

Mr. E avoided eye contact and seemed depressed. When speaking to his children about how he had been faring at his new home, he seemed reluctant to talk about his experiences, causing the children to become even more concerned. His children started visiting more often and encouraging Mr. E with meals and activities. They noticed that he would brighten up when they were together, but toward the end of the visit, he would appear more anxious and depressed. His daughter also noticed that her father seemed especially uncomfortable around one of the staff members. She asked her father directly about his interactions with the staff member. After much reluctance, he stated, "I don't want to make trouble" and revealed that the staff member was very harsh toward him, often berating him with statements such as "You're trying to make my job harder," or even blaming him for malfunctioning equipment.

The family informed the assisted-living facility management, which completed a swift investigation and removed the staff member. Soon after the staff member's dismissal, Mr. E's mood and activities improved. He was more social, eating better, and enjoying the services provided at the assisted-living facility.

Risk Factors of Elder Abuse

When working with older adults, it is important to keep in mind risk factors that make certain individuals more vulnerable to abuse. On the basis of a variety of studies, older adults who are more at risk to be abused share the following characteristics [13].

General Risk Factors

General risk factors include the following:

- Low income or poverty
- Diagnosis of dementia
- Experience of previous traumatic events
- Functional impairments

- Behavioral problems
- Living with a large number of household members
- Low social support

Financial Exploitation

Peterson et al. identified the following factors to be associated with risk of financial exploitation of older adults [23]:

- Nonuse of social services
- Need for assistance in activities of daily living
- Poor self-rated health
- No spouse/partner
- Non-Caucasian older status (in particular this risk was found to be significantly higher among African Americans)

Perpetrators

Though there are limited data, perpetrators are most likely to be as follows [14]:

- Adult children or spouses
- Men
- Socially isolated individuals
- Unemployed or having financial problems
- Experiencing major stress

  They are also more likely to have the following:

- A history of past or current substance abuse
- Mental or physical health problems
- A history of trouble with the police

Assessment of Elder Abuse

Currently, there are no national standards stipulating how clinicians should assess for potential elder abuse. There are a variety of reasons for the absence of standards. These include no widely accepted screening tools, varying definitions of abuse and laws regarding reporting of abuse, and uneasiness of physicians with reporting abuse. Based on these concerns, the US Preventive Services Task Force (USPSTF) concluded that, "The current evidence is insufficient to assess the balance of benefits and harms of screening all elderly or vulnerable adults of abuse and neglect" [29]. However, the USPSTF noted that the potential harm of screening may also be small (shame, fear of retaliation or abandonment by perpetrators, and the repercussions of false-positive results were provided as potential harms). Though the USPSTF does not recommend screening, a number of professional organizations do recommend routine screening. For example, the American Medical Association, which includes elder abuse under the rubric of family violence, recommends that physicians "routinely inquire about the family violence histories of their patients" (AMA Policy Family Violence-Adolescents as Victims and Perpetrators H-515.981).

On the basis of a 2004 review of available screening tools for elder abuse, Fulmer et al. [12] noted that, while there is no one ideal scale, it is important that physicians create a system to implement in their practice. Yaffe et al. [31] recommended the use of the Elder Abuse Suspicion Index, which provides the physician with questions that could raise the concern for elder abuse. It is not a diagnostic tool but one that prompts the physician to enquire about abuse in greater detail. One complicating issue related to assessing for abuse in older adults is the impact of cognitive disorders. Many with cognitive deficits may not be able to provide the information needed during the assessment. While it is commonplace to include family members and caregivers in older-adult care, this, too, may not always be adequate in the setting of elder abuse when the perpetrator is a family member or caregiver, in cases of suspected abuse, it is very important to meet with the patient and family or caregiver separately. Based on a number of recommendations in the literature, questions in Table 11.1 could help identify elder abuse. When asking these questions, it is important to look at nonverbal communications (e.g., eye contact).

TABLE 11.1 Questions to help identify elder abuse

Physical abuse

Has anyone hurt you?

Has anyone threatened you?

Do you feel safe at home?

Psychological/emotional abuse

Has anyone shouted at you?

Has anyone stopped talking to you because they were angry with you?

Do you ever feel alone when your family/caregiver is near?

Has anyone been mean to you?

Do you feel that you will be punished if you disagree with your family/caregiver?

Neglect

Do you have enough food and medications?

When you need something (e.g., clothing, dentures, or eyeglasses), do you have a way of getting it?

Do you have a plan for getting urgent needs met?

Financial abuse

Have you signed any forms that you did not understand?

Have you been forced to sign any forms related to money?

Has access to money or assets been taken away from you?

Sexual abuse

Have you been forced to perform sexual acts against your will?

Do you worry about being sexually violated?

Along with an appropriate history that collects information regarding nutrition, injuries, and treatment adherence, a complete physical examination is critical to assessing for physical abuse. Objective findings of abuse, particularly, physical, sexual, and neglect, can be gleaned from a physical examination. Common findings for physical abuse include injuries to areas that are usually not affected by accidental injuries, e.g., the inner thighs, unexplained fractures, or traumatic alopecia. Sexual abuse may present with intraoral injuries such as that of the palate, vaginal or anorectal bleeding, or injuries secondary to restraints. Neglect can present with unexplained weight loss (inadequate nutrition), poorly controlled medical conditions (nonadherence with medications), or ulcerations in atypical locations, suggesting improper or forced positioning causing undue stress on the musculoskeletal system [5].

Finally, it is important for the examining physician to differentiate common findings in older adults (whether it is because of aging or common medical illnesses) from abuse. Examples include dermatological findings such as senile purpura, nosebleeds and rectal bleeding (from internal hemorrhoids), and dehydration (from reduced thirst sensation).

Interventions for Elder Abuse

Situations in which elder abuse is suspected or identified require the clinician to intervene appropriately. If there are emergent medical situations, for example, acute injuries, serious safety risk, or metabolic instability, immediate inpatient care may be warranted. If possible, clinicians may involve family members or caregivers to devise a safety plan whereby the older adult's health can be safeguarded. As described in later sections in the chapter, healthcare providers also have an obligation to report suspected and identified elder abuse to APS and, possibly, to legal authorities. Depending on the immediate resources available, the medical team can work with the agency and caregivers to create a treatment plan.

Legal Services and Policies

Older Americans Act

The Older Americans Act, passed by Congress in 1965, is a major vehicle for providing support to assist older adults with maintaining their independence in their own homes and communities. Although a large component of the funding is allocated to nutrition and social services such as congregate and home-delivered meals, assistance is also provided for transportation, legal services, caregiver support, community service employment for low-income elderly, training, research, development projects in the field of aging, and vulnerable elder rights protection activities. The Act authorizes service programs to accomplish these tasks through state and Area Agencies on Aging [20]. The Act also established the US Administration on Aging to work closely with Area Agencies on Aging and administer federal programs, such as the National Center on Elder Abuse, which provides elder-abuse awareness and education [3].

Over the years, reauthorization of the Older Americans Act, as recently as 2016, has included provisions that aim to protect vulnerable elders, such as in-home services for the frail elderly; the long-term care ombudsman program; assistance for special needs, health education, and promotion; prevention of elder abuse, neglect, and exploitation; elder rights and legal assistance; and benefits outreach, counseling, and assistance programs [20].

Elder Justice Act

The Elder Justice Act, the first comprehensive legislation to address elder abuse, was signed into law by President Obama on March 23, 2010, as part of the Patient Protection and Affordable Care Act. The aim was to develop and implement strategies to decrease the likelihood of elder abuse, neglect, and exploitation. The Act authorized federal funding for state and local APS programs, support for the Long-Term Care Ombudsman Program, Elder-Abuse Forensic Centers, an Elder Abuse Coordinating Council for federal agencies, and an expert public Advisory Board on Elder Abuse, Neglect and Exploitation, and requires the reporting of crimes in long-term care facilities to law enforcement. At present, Congress has not appropriated funds for the implementation of the Elder Justice Act [18].

Adult Protective Services (APS)

APS are social service agencies that were first formed in the mid-1970s with the passage of Title XX of the Social Security Act [6]. By the early 1980s, every state and/or local government had an agency in its own jurisdiction. APS is responsible for receiving and investigating reports of suspected abuse, neglect, and exploitation. APS staff perform a home visit with the alleged victim, generally within 24–72 hours, to determine whether he or she needs protection and has decision-making capacity to accept or refuse protective services. If warranted, APS will arrange or refer the victim to other services. Other services may include financial management, food or meal delivery, health care, home repair or cleaning, housing (emergency or long term), legal assistance, transportation, and victim assistance and compensation [26]. All states have APS statutes that authorize and regulate provision of services in cases of elder abuse. A few states have both an APS agency and an elder protective service agency that provides services to adults 60 years of age and older [8].

State law governs what types of elder abuse and what categories of victims an APS agency may investigate. State APS statutes may contain eligibility criteria about the following:

- Age: Most states cover persons age 18 years and over, while others cover persons age 60 years and older or 65 years and older.
- Condition: In a majority of states, an individual must have some sort of condition, such as "mental or physical impairment," "mental or physical illness," "mental retardation," "developmental disability," "dementia," or "substance abuse."
- Function: In some states, a person must have impaired ability to do certain things, such as provide self-care; manage finances; protect him/herself; obtain services; or make, communicate, or implement decisions.
- Assistance needed: A few states stipulate that an individual must have no able and willing person available to provide assistance.

- Living situation: In some states, APS will investigate only when a person lives in a house or apartment. Reports made about residents in institutions such as a nursing home are investigated by another agency, such as the long-term care ombudsman program.
- Guardian or conservator: In some states, an individual is automatically eligible for APS if a court has ruled that the person lacks decision-making capacity and has/will appoint a guardian or conservator for that person [26].

A comparison chart [27] on provisions in APS laws by state may be found at: https://www.americanbar.org/content/dam/aba/administrative/law_aging/Abuse_Types_by_State_and_Category_Chart.authcheckdam.pdf

Mandatory Reporting

Most states have a statutory requirement to report elder abuse, neglect, and exploitation. Reporting requirements vary from state to state and are typically in the state's APS laws. In most states, reporting suspected abuse is mandatory for healthcare and social service providers and law enforcement officers. Some states require bankers and other fiduciaries, or any member of the community, to report suspected elder abuse [17]. Failure to report abuse is usually considered a misdemeanor and may be grounds for a fine, imprisonment, loss of license, or other disciplinary action by an employer or a licensing board. Most state APS laws protect the identity of the reporter and provide immunity from criminal, civil, or administrative liability to persons who report abuse or participate in activities stemming from a report [4].

Once APS receives a report, a service specialist conducts an investigation and develops a plan that continues until the case is resolved, or reasonable efforts are made. APS operates under the "least restrictive alternative" philosophy, meaning service specialists identify interventions with the least restrictions on the victims. For example, if an older adult is experiencing difficulty managing his/her finances, someone can make a recommendation for financial counseling. Depending on the situation, a more restrictive option may be needed, for example, to obtain a payee service. In an effort to maintain autonomy and ensure least restrictive alternatives, a victim of abuse may decline APS services if he/she has decision-making capacity [7].

Conclusions

Elder abuse has a fairly high prevalence, despite being under-reported. Given the serious impact of abuse on older adults, clinicians should remain vigilant for warning signs of elder abuse and be knowledgeable of the assessments and interventions necessary to address suspected elder abuse.

References

1. Acierno R, Hernandez MA, Amstadter AB, Resnick HS, Steve K, Muzzy W, et al. Prevalence and correlates of emotional, physical, sexual, and financial abuse and potential neglect in the United States: The National Elder Mistreatment Study. Am J Public Health. 2010;100:292–7. https://doi.org/10.2105/AJPH.2009.163089.
2. American Psychological Association. Elder abuse and neglect: in search of solutions. Washington, DC: Author; 2012. Available from: http://www.apa.org/pi/aging/resources/guides/elder-abuse.pdf.
3. Assistant Secretary for Planning and Evaluation. Performance improvement 2000. Administration on Aging. U.S. Department of Health and Human Services. https://aspe.hhs.gov/report/performance-improvement-2000/administration-aging. Accessed 5 May 2018.
4. Center for Elders and the Courts. Key issues. Mandatory reporting. National Center for State Courts. http://www.ncsc.org/Microsites/CEC/Home/Elder-Abuse/Elder-Abuse-Material-For-Right-Rail-Menu-for-Elder-Abuse/Key-Issues/Mandatory-Reporting.aspx (2018). Accessed 3 May 2018.
5. Collins KA. Elder maltreatment: a review. Arch Pathol Lab Med. 2006;130(9):1290–6.
6. Department of Family and Protective Services Texas Adult Protective Services (APS). n.d. https://www.dfps.state.tx.us/Adult_Protection/. Accessed 8 May 2018.

7. Department of Family and Protective Services. Adult protective services handbook. n.d. https://www.state.tx.us/handbooks/APS/Files/APS_pg_3200.asp. Accessed 8 May 2018.

8. Department of Health and Human Services Aging & Disability Services Division. Elder protective services. 2017.

9. Dong X, Simon M, de Leon CM, Fulmer T, Beck T, Hebert L, et al. Elder self-neglect and abuse and mortality risk in a community-dwelling population. JAMA. 2009;302:517–26. https://doi.org/10.1001/jama.2009.1109.

10. Eckroth-Bucher M. Devious damage: elder psychological abuse. 2008. http://www.todaysgeriatricmedicine.com/archive/101308p24.shtml. Accessed 6 Feb 2018.

11. Elder Abuse. n.d. https://www.cdc.gov/violenceprevention/elder-abuse/definitions.html. Accessed 27 June 2018.

12. Fulmer T, Guadagno L, Dyer CB, Connolly MT. Progress in elder abuse screening and assessment instruments. J Am Geriatr Soc. 2004;52:297–304. https://doi.org/10.1111/j.1532-5415.2004.52074.x.

13. Johannesen M, Lo Giudice D. Elder abuse: a systematic review of risk factors in community-dwelling elders. Age Ageing. 2013;42(3):292–8. https://doi.org/10.1093/ageing/afs195.

14. Lachs MS, Pillemer KA. Elder abuse. N Engl J Med. 2015;373:1947–56. https://doi.org/10.1056/NEJMra1404688.

15. National Adult Protective Services Association. Elder financial exploitation.n.d. http://www.napsa-now.org/policy-advocacy/exploitation/. Accessed 21 Nov 2017.

16. National Adult Protective Services Association. Get informed. Other safety concerns and self-neglect. n.d. http://www.napsa-now.org/get-informed/other-safety-concerns-2/. Accessed 16 Nov 2017.

17. National Adult Protective Services Association. How APS helps. 2018a. http://www.napsa-now.org/get-help/how-aps-helps/. Accessed 8 May 2018.

18. National Adult Protective Services Association (NAPSA). Elder Justice Act. 2018b. http://www.napsa-now.org/policy-advocacy/eja-implementation/. Accessed 5/3/18.

19. National Center on Elder Abuse. Attitudes toward elder mistreatment and reporting: a multicultural study. Washington DC: National Center on Elder Abuse; 1998.

20. National Committee to Preserve Social Security and Medicare. Older Americans Act. Government relations and policy. 2016. https://www.ncpssm.org/documents/older-americans-policy-papers/older-americans-act/.Accessed 27 June 2018.

21. National Institute on Aging. Elder Abuse. Last updated December 29, 2016. n.d. http://www.nia.nih.gov/health/elder-abuse. Accessed 21 Nov 2017.

22. Ortman JM, Velkoff VA, Hogan H. An aging nation: the older population in the United States. Population estimates and projections. Current Population Reports. 2014 (May)/P25–1140. https://www.census.gov/prod/2014pubs/p25-1140.pdf. Accessed 20 Mar 2018.

23. Peterson JC, Burnes DP, Caccamise PL, Mason A, Henderson CJ, Wells MT, et al. Financial exploitation of older adults: a population-based prevalence study. J Gen Intern Med. 2014;29:1615–23. https://doi.org/10.1007/s11606-014-2946-2.

24. Pillemer K, Burnes D, Riffin C, Lachs MS. Elder abuse: global situation, risk factors, and prevention strategies. Gerontologist. 2016;56:S194–205. https://doi.org/10.1093/geront/gnw00410.1093/geront/gnw004.

25. Smith AK, Lo B, Aronson L. Elder self-neglect — how can a physician help? N Engl J Med. 2013;369:2476–9. https://doi.org/10.1056/NEJMp1310684doi:10.1056/NEJMp1310684.

26. Stiegel L. Legal issues related to elder abuse: a desk guide for law enforcement. American Bar Association Commission on Law and Aging. 2015. https://www.americanbar.org/content/dam/aba/administrative/law_aging/ABAElderAbuseDeskGuide.auth-checkdam.pdf. Accessed 3 May 2018.

27. Stiegel L, Klem E. Types of abuse: comparison chart of provisions in adult protective services laws, by State. American Bar Association. 2007. long-term care ombudsman program. Accessed 26 June 2018.

28. Teaster PB, Roberto KA. Sexual abuse of older adults: APS cases and outcomes. Gerontologist. 2004;44:788–96. https://doi.org/10.1093/geront/44.6.788.

29. U.S. Preventive Services Task Force. Understanding Task Force recommendations. Screening for intimate partner violence and abuse of elderly and vulnerable adults. Final Recommendation; 2013.

30. World Health Organization, University of Toronto and Ryerson University, The International Network for the Prevention of Elder Abuse. The Toronto declaration on the global prevention of elder abuse. Geneva: World Health Organization; 2002.

31. Yaffe MJ, Wolfson C, Lithwick M, Weiss D. Development and validation of a tool to improve physician identification of elder abuse: the elder abuse suspicion index (EASI). J Elder Abuse Negl. 2008;20(3):276–300. https://doi.org/10.1080/08946560801973168.

Part III
Forensic Aspects
of Geriatric Psychiatry

Chapter 12
Social Determinants and Mental Health Among Older Adults in the Criminal Justice System

Tina Maschi and Dhweeja Dasarathy

Background

The case vignettes of Grace, Edgar, and Diego illustrated in Table 12.1 only scratch the surface of the rapidly growing global aging and mental health crisis, particularly in United States' prisons. Of the approximate 2.6 million people in United States' prisons as of 2010, about 220,000 (16%) were aged 50 and older [1]. The Bureau of Justice Statistics (BJA) reported that in the past two decades the state prison population aged 55 and older has increased from 3% (1993) to 10% [2]. This increase has largely been attributed to the growing

T. Maschi (✉)
Fordham University Graduate School of Social Service,
New York, NY, USA
e-mail: tmaschi@fordham.edu

D. Dasarathy
Harvard University, Cambridge, MA, USA
e-mail: ddsarathy@college.harvard.edu

© Springer Nature Switzerland AG 2019   185
M. Balasubramaniam et al. (eds.), *Psychiatric Ethics in Late-Life Patients*, https://doi.org/10.1007/978-3-030-15172-0_12

TABLE 12.1 Case vignettes

Grace: Grace is a 58-year-old, Caucasian, Catholic woman with a high school diploma and a history of steady employment. She is serving a 10-year prison sentence in a maximum-security women's prison. As a child, she experienced the divorce of her parents, abandonment by her mother, and physical and verbal abuse by her father, whom she described as having serious mental health problems. At age 23, Grace reported she married a man 6 years younger, had two children, and divorced him after 7 years of marriage. At intake, she told her prison psychiatrist that this is her first and only criminal conviction and she is serving a 10-year prison sentence for conspiracy to commit murder of her husband. Grace described her sentence as "unfair and unjust" based on the mitigating circumstances of domestic violence victimization. While in prison, she was diagnosed with post-traumatic stress and major depressive disorders and was prescribed the anti-depressant medication, fluoxetine, by the prison psychiatrist. Prior to prison, her medical history included hypertension and arthritis with associated chronic neck and shoulder pain. At age 58, Grace's extensive dental problems also have resulted in a premature need for dentures. She described her current prison experience as "neglectful, especially the lack of health accessibility to prison mental health and health services." Grace's projected parole date is in 2 years, when she will be 60 years old. Grace noted plans to cope with her prison experience by "finding meaning" in the experience through spirituality. She also reported she would like to visit with her two children. However, she has been unable to connect with the prison case manager/social worker to help arrange these in-person or video conference visits.

Edgar: Edgar is a 60-year-old, bisexual, African American male with a history of homelessness and mental illness (schizophrenia) and reported having no high school diploma. He reported having had a "nervous breakdown" because he "lost everything," including his job and apartment. Two years later, in a drunken rage, he "broke the law" and spent 1 year in a county jail. After his release, he reports being unable to obtain basic needs, such as food, water, clothing, housing, and healthcare. He was reluctant to seek assistance from family and friends, social services, or church due to shame and embarrassment. He reported that he subsequently committed a crime for the purpose of returning to prison where he felt his basic needs would more easily be met. Edgar also reported improvement in his ability to cope because he was prescribed psychotropic medication (Haldol) and received one-on-one counseling with a prison social worker. While in prison, he also was diagnosed with diabetes and asthma. He also reported, while in prison, that he had minimal family contact and was ongoingly being harassed by younger inmates. Edgar is expecting to be released from prison in 1–2 years if approved by the parole board.

Diego: Diego is a 62-year-old Puerto Rican male and the youngest of 12 children. He reported being a high school dropout, a victim of childhood trauma such as the unexpected death of his father at age 6, sexual victimization (by an aunt), growing up in poverty, engaging in teenage prostitution and drug dealing as a young adult, opioid addiction, and he reported committing armed robbery to support his opioid addiction, and he was sentenced to a mandatory 25-year sentence. During his prison term, he reported his continued use of illicit drugs that were smuggled into the prison. After his first prison release, he violated parole within 12 months. As a result, he is now serving his second and current 20-year to 50-year sentence. In prison, he has spent 8 of his first 15 years in solitary confinement because of his violent behavior when housed in general population. Since, he has received several disciplinary infractions for aggressive and violent behavior while placed in general prison population. During an appointment with the prison psychiatrist, Diego described prison as "an overcrowded monster" designed to hold, degrade, and punish people. He was diagnosed with post-traumatic stress disorder positively associated with spending a significant amount of time in solitary confinement. He also said he was upset about the mental health and correctional staff as disinterested and disengaged. He also reported feeling despondent over the limited access to counseling and education rehabilitative services. Although he was prescribed psychotropic medication, he has not been compliant with taking his medication or attending prison programs, such as anger or stress management. He also reported he has not had any family visits in over 10 years.

segment of incarcerated people who are aged 55+ serving long-term prison sentences, mostly for serious violent offenses. Official statistics also suggest that as many as half of adults aged 50 and older in prison are diagnosed with some type of mental health problem, including serious mental illnesses, such as major depression, schizophrenia, and cognitive impairments, such as dementia [3]. Available evidence also suggests that there is a subpopulation of older adults with histories of minor to serious mental illnesses and co-occurring addiction. The types of disorders noted among current studies include post-traumatic stress disorder, substance abuse disorders, major depressive disorders, dementia, and schizophrenia, in the criminal justice system, especially among older adults in prison, as highlighted in the three case vignettes [4, 5].

Evidence also suggests that there is a biological process of accelerated aging among older people in prison that also influences their mental health status. That is, people in prison tend to age 10–15 years faster than their community counterparts. This process may be an after product of their high-risk personal histories or social determinants of health (e.g., homelessness, poverty, substance use, poor diet, and lack of access to health services). Their health conditions are further exacerbated by the stressful conditions of confinement that include exposure to violence, overcrowding, and poor environmental conditions (e.g., lack of fresh air, adequate lighting, malnutrition, dehydration, and lack of access to quality health and mental health services while in prison) [6–8].

Due to the fact that mental and physical health problems are intertwined among incarcerated older adults that intersect with social determinants of health, such as employment, family, housing, social security, and financial assistance, it is imperative that there is an integrated and interdisciplinary response to address the mental health and social structural issues impacting this vulnerable population of older adults. To this end, this chapter provides an overview of mental health issues, including the social determinants of mental health, among older people involved in the criminal justice system, particularly who are serving sentences in prison. It incorporates case vignettes and evidence from the peer-reviewed literature to highlight the mental health and social environmental treatment issues that practitioners, often in interprofessional teams, commonly addressed when working with older adults with behavioral health problems in the criminal justice system.

Mental Health Assessment and Intervention

There is a growing body of empirical literature that targets the mental health of older people involved in the criminal justice system. In total, we located 44 peer-reviewed journal articles published between 1980 and 2018 that addressed aging, mental health, criminality, and/or the criminal justice system. The majority of the articles most commonly documented the prevalence of serious mental health illnesses, such as schizophrenia, major depressive disorder, and dementia, particularly among older adults who came in contact with the courts, prisons, and psychiatric hospitals for committing alleged or being convicted of one or more criminal offenses. For example, several studies found that older adults who were diagnosed with dementia were more likely to be detected in early in the criminal justice trajectory, particularly prior to a court trial as opposed to jails or prisons [9, 10].

Many of the studies documented evidence of serious mental illnesses among the aging prison population. For example, older adults with schizophrenia in the criminal justice system represented anywhere from 2% to 91% of a criminal justice setting and were primarily housed in forensic psychiatric hospitals/units inside a correctional system. As for major depressive disorder, most older adults were commonly diagnosed with this mood disorder after they were in a prison setting. Interestingly, there was a significant unexplored research and practice gap in the literature about justice-involved older adults with respect to the prevalence of other common mental health disorders found among the general criminal justice population, such as post-traumatic stress disorder, anxiety, dissociation, suicide risk, and co-occurring substance abuse and other addictions. As clearly illustrated by Grace, Edgar, and Diego profiles, their psychosocial histories show the presence and influence of cumulative traumatic events, such as sexual and physical victimization, family and community violence, went undetected and untreated for most of their lives and challenged their psychological, emotional, social, and behavioral well-being. In addition, prior life history events were exacerbated by stress related to the trauma of incarceration, especially Diego who spent 8 years in solitary confinement.

In order to address this gap, conducting comprehensive mental health assessments for all possible disorders among older adults commonly found among a younger justice population is warranted. For example, in addition to assessing for serious mental illness, other possible associated traumatic stress disorders, mood disorders related to anxiety and depression, personality disorders associated with trauma histories, such as borderline personality disorder, and addictions (e.g., alcohol, drug, nicotine, gambling) should also be assessed. Additionally, the incorporation of a detailed biopsychosocial assessment, often prepared by a social worker, also can assist with identifying many of the historical and current social environmental risk and protective factors that will have an influence on the mental and overall well-being of justice-involved older adults. A comprehensive mental health assessment could be particularly useful in the case of Diego to assess the impact of his long-term placement in solitary confinement.

In addition to assessing for the "mental health problem," the literature also underscored the importance that when older adults are in contact with the criminal justice system, there is increased access to mental health treatment and other related services. Several studies found that the use of comprehensive mental health assessments significantly increased the use of referrals for older adults to receive mental health services whether it be in the courts, jails, or prisons. For example, studies of court settings were often of assessment of older adults' competency to stand trial or increasing referrals or diverting them to mental health services. Prison studies also found that most older adults diagnosed with serious mental illnesses, such as schizophrenia or dementia or personality disorders, were more likely to be referred for psychiatric care, including transfer to forensic psychiatric units [11–13]. As illustrated in the case vignettes of Grace, Edgar, and Diego who were diagnosed with serious mental health issues, all three would benefit from referral and access to psychiatric follow-up and individual and group mental health treatment while in prison and post prison release.

Social Determinants of Mental Health and Criminal Justice Involvement

In addition to providing mental health services "as usual" to justice-involved older adults, it is equally as important to link them to wraparound services that address the common social determinants of these mental health among older adults in the justice system. Research studies on justice-involved older adults have generated empirical evidence for social determinants of mental health that include gender/race (e.g., a higher risk for males and racial ethnic minorities), histories of earlier onset or prolonged mental illness, prior access to mental health assessment and treatment, housing status (e.g., history of homelessness or solitary confinement), education and employment history, the frequency, magnitude, and duration of past interpersonal trauma and chronic stress (i.e., life course cumulative trauma), level of family and social support, spirituality/religious practices, and criminal justice history [11, 14–16]. As illustrated in the case studies of Grace, Edgar, and Diego, the accumulation of social determinants of mental health (e.g., trauma and stress histories, low levels of education, access to mental health and social services) was described by them as a risk factor for the onset of prolonged mental health issues, criminal behavior, and justice system involvement. On the other hand, religion and spirituality were found to be an important protective factor among older adults in prison [17, 18]. For example, Koenig (1995) found that older adults who reported being raised by someone with a religious affiliation were significantly associated with lower depressive symptoms [18]. The study also found that incarcerated older adults who reported attending religious services more frequently reported lower levels of depressive symptoms that attended less frequently [18]. Allen (2008) also found that for older male inmates in Alabama, having a greater number of daily spiritual experiences and religion was associated with better emotional health [17]. As in the case example of Grace, she was naturally drawn to practicing spirituality to find meaning in her life and prison experiences. Given the importance of these social determinants (risk/protective factors) for mental well-being among justice-involved older adults, we have incorporated them in the next section, case application, as part of a comprehensive intervention plan for justice-involved older adults.

Case Application

Consistent with the literature, Grace, Edgar, and Diego reported many of the common psychosocial issues experienced by a rapidly growing population of older adults with mental health issues involved in the criminal justice system. It also is an expanding practice arena for forensic psychiatrists, psychologists, social workers, lawyers, and other interdisciplinary professionals to become more competent in providing geriatric forensic mental health services to this vulnerable older special population. Perhaps most important is to adopt a team-oriented approach to collaborate across disciplines to address the compendium of the root causes and mental health consequences of the social determinants of mental health. As illustrated in the cases of Grace, Edgar, and Diego, the presence of serious mental health issues, such as schizophrenia and major depression, and other common mental health issues, such as post-traumatic stress disorder, is commonly part of the mental health case load, especially for forensic psychiatrists, psychologists, clinical social workers, and case managers (social workers or nurses). In addition to the use of the DSM 5 for mental health assessment, Table 12.2 provides examples of a battery of assessment tools that can be used to assess for commonly found mental health issues among the justice-involved aging population [19]. These

TABLE 12.2 Recommendation for assessment tools for intake and treatment monitoring

Traumatic and Stressful Life Experiences. Trauma and stressful life experiences (cumulative objective occurrences and past year subjective distress) will be measured using the 31-item Life Stressors Checklist-Revised (LSC-R). The LSC-R estimates the frequency of the objective occurrences of lifetime and current traumatic events (e.g., being a victim of and/or witness to violence. The LSC-R has good psychometric properties, including use with diverse age groups and criminal justice populations [29].

Mental Health Symptoms. Mental health symptoms can be measured: Diagnostic and Statistical Manual 5 [20] and the Brief Symptom Inventory (BSI). Subscales include Somatization, Obsessive-Compulsive, Interpersonal Sensitivity, Depression, Anxiety, Hostility, Phobic Anxiety. Paranoid Ideation, Psychoticism [22]

Post-traumatic Stress Symptoms. Post-traumatic stress symptoms were measured with the PTSD Checklist (PCL) for civilian populations [28].

Coping Resources. Coping resources were measured using the Coping Resources Inventory (CRI) [25]. The CRI is a valid measure of self-reported coping resources that are available to manage stressors and has been used with samples of older adults and criminal offenders. This 60-item CRI has five subscales that measure cognitive, emotional, spiritual and philosophical, physical, and social coping resources.

Activities of Daily Living. The Katz Index of Independence in Activities of Daily Living, commonly referred to as the Katz ADL, is the most proper scale to assess functional status as a measurement of an individual's ability to perform activities of daily living independently. Although no formal reliability and validity reports could be found in the literature, the tool is used extensively as a flag, signaling functional capabilities of older adults in clinical and home environments [24].

Geriatric Depression Scale. Geriatric Depression Scale (GDS) is a self-report measure of depression in older adults and also assesses for suicidal risk. The GDS has been used with older prison populations [30].

(continued)

TABLE 12.2 (continued)

Montreal Cognitive Assessment: The Montreal Cognitive Assessment was used to assess for cognitive impairment [27].

Substance Abuse/Addictions: The Addiction Severity Index is a semi-structured instrument used in face-to-face interviews conducted by clinicians, researchers, or trained technicians. The ASI covers the following areas: medical, employment/support, drug and alcohol use, legal, family/social, and psychiatric. The ASI obtains lifetime information about problem behaviors, as well as problems within the previous 30 days [26].

Risk and Needs Assessments/Discharge Planning: (1) Correctional Offender Management and Profiling Alternative Sanctions (COMPAS) assesses needs and risk of recidivism (general recidivism, violent recidivism, noncompliance, and failure to appear). (2) Level of Service Inventory–Revised [21] assesses parole outcome, success in correctional halfway houses, institutional misconducts, and recidivism. (3) *For individuals with sexual offense histories:* The Static-99 is a 10-item actuarial assessment instrument for use with adult sexual offenders who are 18 years or older at the time of community release [23].

assessment tools can be incorporated as a routine assessment to identify mental health issues in the early to late stages of criminal justice involvement to inform practice decision-making. Strengthening early mental health detection mechanisms also may prevent the pathways to many older adults being placed from prison settings to more appropriate settings, such as specialized geriatric or mental health units in prison or community forensic mental health services or psychiatric hospitals after their release.

In addition to access to mental health assessment and services for incarcerated older adults, such as Grace, Edgar, and Diego, interventions that address their social determinants of mental health, such as access to housing, employment, education, and social supports while also in mental health treatment, are important to provide services for them. Based on the case histories, the risk factors, such as untreated childhood traumas, poverty, and lack of access to steady employment or services, placed these individuals at risk for criminal justice involvement, including recidivism. For example, in the case of Edgar, he readily admits to committing a crime in order to return to prison to access housing, food, and mental health and health services. Similarly, in the case of Grace, she reported a history of parental abandonment and abuse and domestic violence victimization as an adult. It was not until prison when Grace had access to mental health services that she could begin managing her mental health symptoms. In the case of Diego, he reported that severe childhood trauma, particularly sexual victimization and living in poverty, has had a lingering effect on his mental/behavioral well-being. In Diego's case, a case manager might assess the extent to whether moving him from the general prison population (where he is at risk of getting placed in solitary confinement again) to a secure mental health in patient unit might be warranted.

In addition to mental treatment, case management services for reentry planning are relevant to Grace and Edgar, who are poised to be released on parole in 1–2 years. In both of their cases, access to discharge planning, social workers, and/or nurses to identify what social determinants need to be in place for their successful reentry process, such as access to safe housing (e.g., home place placement, assisted living or skill nursing facilities), education, employment, social service, trauma or substance abuse assessment and treatment, and assist them to connect with these needed services can be advantageous. In a team-based approach, professionals such as forensic psychiatrists and psychologists can provide referrals and treatment. In the case of Edgar, if he had access to a case manager in the community who connected him with available community services after his first incarceration, it may have decreased his risk of committing a crime to obtain housing, food, and mental health treatment.

It also is recommended that forensic professionals advocate across criminal justice settings (e.g., the courts, prisons) to incorporate comprehensive mental health assessments and interventions (as illustrated in Tables 12.2 and 12.3). Table 12.3 provides an overview of possible interventions that might comprise a comprehensive intervention plan that is relevant to justice-involved older adults, including Grace, Edgar, and Diego. Table 12.4 illustrates a comprehensive intervention

TABLE 12.3 Possible Program Activities

1. *Referrals or Consults.* Self- or staff-generated referrals to psychiatrist or clinical staff for mental health and other services.

2. *Education and Vocational Training and Employment.* Access to a range of vocational services to obtain General Educational Development (GED) or high school diplomas, college degrees, and vocational training in occupations, such as the culinary arts and select trades. Assistance to access to employment while in prison or post reentry.

3. *Recreational Activities.* Arts-based diversion activities. These activities may include crocheting, knitting, beading, and latch-hook rug-making. These activities are not only cognitively stimulating, but also afford excellent physical therapy for arthritic hands and fingers

4. *Culturally Responsive Cognitive Interventions.* Cognitive interventions include creative writing, Spanish language study group, ethnodrama, and cultural arts group. The groups produce a newsletter and poetry journal, which are edited by the group members.

5. *Mental Health, Substance Abuse/Addiction Services: Individual.* Weekly or biweekly visits with prison mental health staff, including psychiatrist for psychotropic medication, psychologists for ongoing evaluations, and social workers for individual clinical treatment (including medication management), and social work and/or nursing case management/discharge planning specialists.

6. *Mental Health, Substance Abuse/Addiction Services: Groups.* Weekly meetings of 12-step groups, including Alcoholics Anonymous, Narcotics Anonymous, and Sexual Compulsives Anonymous, grief and bereavement, trauma which may be facilitated by trained professionals (prison staff or community volunteers) or trained peers in prison (when appropriate), including anger and stress management and sex offense or violent offense group treatment.

7. *Medical Services.* Assistance with access to prison and community medical services in a timely fashion. Ongoing monitoring of serious and/or chronic health conditions. In the case of terminal illnesses, referrals for end-of-life care.

8. *Physical and Psycho-education.* Weekly seminars to address prison adjustment, psychosocial well-being, address aging, health and wellness, sexuality, life skills, cooking, menu-planning, financial and retirement planning, and healthy life choices, or other relevant activities. Weekly exercise programs to maintain health and well-being.

9. *Restorative Justice/Reconciliation and Forgiveness Groups/Long-termers and Lifers Group.* Access to special groups for reconciliation and forgiveness. These groups often use narrative-style writing and group reflection for individuals to process their crime, especially violent or sexual offenses that resulted in the harm or death to another person or persons. For participants with life sentences, a weekly lifers group is offered.

10. *Animal-Assisted Therapy.* Animal-assisted therapy (individually and in group) that targets physical, occupational, speech and psychotherapies, special education, pain management issues, and end of life support.

11. *Prison Legal Services and Victims' Rights Training.* Prison legal services program participants' access to pro bono lawyers and social workers who are versed in elder and prison rights and law and case management services. Program participants can seek consultation or representation for appeals based on sentencing, parole release, or geriatric, medical, and compassionate release. The prison Ombudsman represents cases of interpersonal victimization and institutional abuse. Community advocates who monitor cases based on the Prison Rape Elimination Act also are available to incarcerated persons at the facility, including program participants.

12. *Family/Peer Volunteer Visiting Programs (in-person or televisiting).* Access to family visiting programs that provide extended time with family members, which includes spouses and partners, children, and grandchildren. Families can request transportation services from faith-based volunteers if there is no access to public transportation to get to the facility. An option for televisiting was available for participants, such as Mary, whose family lived at a distance that did not enable them to visit her in person. For participants without family members who can visit, peer visits and volunteer visitors can be arranged based on request.

13. *Case Management/Discharge Planning/Reentry Preparedness.* Access to case management services while in prison and/or preparing for release. Assistance by trained medical and social service professionals or trained peer support staff while in prison and/or the community. Access to information and referrals, especially related to Medicare or Medicaid and other documentation needed post release, referrals to collaborating agencies, such as nonprofit organizations, halfway houses, resources for potential housing, employment, social security and other benefits, and other assistance.

TABLE 12.4 Intervention plan for case vignettes

Intervention plan	Grace	Edgar	
Treatment Goals	1. Increase mental health and overall well-being. 2. Increase preparedness for community reintegration.	1. Increase mental health and overall well-being. 2. Increase preparedness for community reintegration.	1. Increase mental health and overall well-being. 2. Reduce disciplinary infractions to zero.
Possible interventions			
Referrals and/ or consults for mental health or other services	X	X	X
Educational and vocational training	X	X	X
Recreational activities	X	X	X
Culturally responsive cognitive interventions	X	X	X
Mental health/ Addictions services- individual (professional)	X	X	X
Mental health/ Addictions services-group (professional/ peer)	X	X	X

TABLE 12.4 (continued)

Intervention plan	Grace	Edgar	
Medical services	X	X	X
Physical and psycho-education	X	X	X
Animal-assisted therapy		X	
Family, volunteer, or peer visiting program	X	X	X
Spiritual wellness	X	X	
Prisoner legal services & victim rights services	X	X	X
Family/peer/ volunteer visiting program	X	X	X
Education and vocational training	X	X	x
Case management (while in prison)	X	X	X
Discharge planning (release preparation)	X	X	X

plan for Grace, Edgar, and Diego. On a final note, community placement challenges for these three cases with violent and/ or sexual offense histories often are more challenging to obtain basic needs post release. In many cases, case managers often must educate and advocate on older adults' behalf [15].

Conclusion

In summary, this chapter provided an overview of mental health issues, including the social determinants of mental health, commonly found among justice-involved older adults. We asserted throughout this chapter that effective mental health assessment and treatment must be comprehensive and target the social determinants of mental health. Interdisciplinary professionals can play a key role in developing and refining innovative mental health/criminal justice programs for older people and their families and communities. For examples of existing programs for justice-involved older adults, please see the following chapter.

References

1. At America's expense: the mass incarceration of the elderly [Internet]. American Civil Liberties Union. [cited 17 Aug 2018]. Available from: https://www.aclu.org/americas-expense-mass-incarceration-elderly.
2. Carson EA, Sabol WJ. Aging of the state prison population, 1993–2013. Washington D.C.: U.S. Department of Justice, Office of Justice Programs.
3. James D, Glaze L. Mental health problems of prison and jail inmates. Washington D.C.: U.S. Department of Justice, Office of Justice Programs; 2006.
4. Arndt S, Turvey C, Flaum M. Older offenders, substance abuse, and treatment. Am J Geriatr Psychiatry. 2002;10:733–9.
5. Murdoch N, Morris P, Holmes C. Depression in elderly life sentence prisoners. Int J Geriatr Psychiatry. 2008;23(9):957–62.
6. Anno BJ, Graham C, Lawrence J, Shansky R. Addressing the needs of elderly, chronically ill, and terminally ill inmates. Middletown: Criminal Justice Inc.

7. Old Behind Bars | The aging prison population in the United States [Internet]. Human Rights Watch. 2016 [cited Aug]. Available from: http://www.hrw.org/reports/2012/01/27/old-behind-bars

8. Wilson J, Barboza S. The looming challenge of dementia in corrections. PsycEXTRA Dataset. 2010.

9. Frierson R, Shea SJ, Shea MEC. Competence-to-stand-trial evaluations of geriatric defendants. J Am Acad Psychiatry Law. 2002;30:252–6.

10. Lewis CF, Fields C, Rainey E. A study of geriatric forensic evaluees: who are the violent elderly? J Am Acad Psychiatry Law. 2006 Sep;34(3)

11. Curtice M, Parker J, Wismayer FS, Tomison A. The elderly offender: an 11-year survey of referrals to a regional forensic psychiatric service. J Forensic Psychiatry Psychol. 2003;14(2):253–65.

12. Heinik J, Kimhi R, Hes JP. Dementia and crime: a forensic psychiatry unit study in Israel. Int J Geriatr Psychiatry. 1994;9(6):491–4.

13. Shah A. An audit of a specialist old age psychiatry liaison service to a medium and a high secure forensic psychiatry unit. Med Sci Law. 2006;46(2):99–104.

14. Farragher B, Oconnor A. Forensic psychiatry and elderly people — a retrospective review. Med Sci Law. 1995;35(3):269–73.

15. Maschi T, Viola D, Koskinen L. Trauma, stress, and coping among older adults in prison: towards a human rights and intergenerational family justice action agenda. Traumatology. 2015;21(3):188–200.

16. Haugebrook S, Zgoba KM, Maschi T, Morgen K, Brown D. Trauma, stress, health, and mental health issues among ethnically diverse older adult prisoners. J Correct Health Care. 2010;16(3):220–9.

17. Allen RS, Phillips LL, Roff LL, Cavanaugh R, Day L. Religiousness/spirituality and mental health among older male inmates. The Gerontologist. 2008;48(5):692–7.

18. Koenig HG. Religion and older men in prison. Int J Geriatr Psychiatry. 1995;10(3):219–30.

19. Diagnostic and statistical manual of mental disorders: DSM-5. Arlington: American Psychiatric Association; 2013.

20. American Psychiatric Association. Diagnostic and statistical manual of mental disorders. 5th ed. Arlington: American Psychiatric Publishing; 2013.

21. Andrews DA, Bonta J. LSI-R: The level of service inventory–revised. Toronto: Multi-Health Systems, Inc; 1995.
22. Derogatis L. Brief symptom inventory manual. Boston: Pearson Publishers; 1993.
23. Hanson K, Babchishin K, Helmus L, Thornton D. Quantifying the relative risk of sex offenders., Risk ratios for Static 99-R. Sexual Abuse A Journal of Research and Treatment. 2013;25:482–515.
24. Katz S, Akpom CA. 12. Index of ADL. Medical Care. 1976;14(5):116–8.
25. Marting MS, Hammer AL. Coping Resources Inventory manual-revised. Menlo: Mind Garden, Inc; 2004.
26. Martino S. Addiction severity index. In: Fisher G, Roget N, editors. Encyclopedia of substance abuse prevention, treatment, & recovery. Thousand Oaks, CA: SAGE Publications, Inc; 2009. p. 15–7.
27. Nasreddine ZS, Phillips NA, Bédirian V, Charbonneau S, Whitehead V, Collin I, et al. The Montreal Cognitive Assessment (MoCA): a brief screening tool for mild cognitive impairment. Journal of the American Geriatrics Society. 2005;53:695–699, 2005.
28. Weathers FW, Litz BT, Herman DS, Huska JA, Keane TM. The PTSD checklist: Reliability, validity, and diagnostic utility. Paper presented at the annual meeting of the International Society for Traumatic Stress Studies, San Antonio, 1993.
29. Wolfe JW, Kimerling R, Brown PJ, Chrestman KR, Levin K. Psychometric review of the Life Stressor Checklist-Revised. In: Stamm BH, editor. Measurement of stress, trauma, and adaptation. Lutherville, Sidran Press; 1996. p. 31–53.
30. Yesavage JA, Brink TL, Rose TL, Lum O, Huang V, Adey M, Leirer VO. Development and validation of a geriatric depression screening scale: a preliminary report. Journal of Psychiatric Research. 1983;17:37–49.

Chapter 13
Capacity to Stand Trial Evaluations for Geriatric Defendants

Monika Pietrzak, Jeremy Colley, and Bipin Subedi

Legal Standard for Competency to Stand Trial as Determined by Judicial Rulings

Courts in the United States, via a series of cases, have defined the legal standard by which a defendant facing criminal charges is competent to stand trial. Similar to evaluation of competence to make treatment decisions with regard to medical care, defendants, in the abstract, must be able to understand and retain information relevant to the decision in question, apply that understanding to their specific circumstances in the context of their individual values, and reason

———
M. Pietrzak
New York University School of Medicine, New York, NY, USA
e-mail: Monika.Pietrzak2@nyulangone.org

J. Colley · B. Subedi (✉)
Department of Psychiatry, New York University School of
Medicine, New York, NY, USA
e-mail: Jeremy.colley@nyumc.org; Bipin.subedi@nyumc.org

© Springer Nature Switzerland AG 2019   203
M. Balasubramaniam et al. (eds.), *Psychiatric Ethics in
Late-Life Patients*, https://doi.org/10.1007/978-3-030-15172-0_13

among options available to them. The Supreme Court has more precisely defined the contours of these general elements of competence for a criminal defendant through a series of legal decisions, the first of which was *Dusky v. U.S.*[1].

Milton Dusky was charged with kidnapping a 15-year-old girl and transporting her across state lines. The girl was raped by Dusky's two juvenile accomplices (aged 14 and 16 years), one of whom was tried separately and convicted as an adult. Dusky's attorney raised issues of insanity and incompetence to stand trial, and the Court ordered a psychiatric examination. Evaluating psychiatrists attested that Dusky suffered from chronic undifferentiated schizophrenia, experienced hallucinations and delusions about being framed, and was unable to meet reality demands. In a competency report provided to the trial court, an expert psychiatrist contended that Dusky was unable to properly understand the proceedings and could not adequately assist counsel in his defense. Despite this testimony, the trial judge ruled that Dusky was competent to stand trial because he was oriented and appeared to understand the nature of the charges against him.

Dusky was convicted and sentenced to 45 years. He appealed, asserting that the trial court erred in finding him competent to stand trial.

The Supreme Court reversed Dusky's conviction, identifying competence to stand trial as a fundamental constitutional right, and citing insufficient evidence to support the district court's decision that he was competent to stand trial. The Court concluded that it was not enough for a defendant to be oriented to time and place and to have some recollection of events, and articulated a two-prong test as the minimum Constitutional standard by which a defendant must be found competent to stand trial. Specifically, they indicated that competence to stand trial hinges on "whether [the defendant] has sufficient present ability to consult with his lawyer with a reasonable degree of rational understanding – and whether he has a rational as well as factual understanding of the proceedings against him." This definition of adjudicative competence is commonly known as the *Dusky* standard. Notably, the opinion did not provide guidance on how to practically apply these prongs; instead, it left such competency determinations to be decided by trial courts based on the particular facts of the case at hand.

The case was remanded for a hearing to determine Dusky's present competency, and for a new trial if he was found to be competent, using the standard articulated by the Supreme Court.

In *Drope v. Missouri,* building upon its earlier decision in *Dusky*, the Supreme Court proclaimed that a trial court must always be alert to circumstances that would render the defendant incompetent [2]. Furthermore, the trial court has an independent duty to request a competency evaluation whenever evidence raises "sufficient doubt" as to the defendant's competence.

James Drope was charged with forcibly raping his wife. His attorney filed a pretrial motion for a continuance so that Drope could receive psychiatric evaluation and treatment. The motion was supported by a psychiatric report, which outlined Drope's mental health issues and corroborated the need for psychiatric treatment. The trial court denied the motion and directed the case to proceed to trial. Drope's wife testified about her husband's history of irrational behaviors and his attempt to choke her shortly before the start of trial. The next morning, Drope unsuccessfully attempted suicide. Defense counsel then requested a mistrial based on his client's required hospitalization. However, the trial court concluded that Drope waived his right to be present because his inability to appear stemmed from a voluntary act and ordered the trial to continue in his absence.

Drope was convicted in absentia and sentenced to life imprisonment. On appeal, he asserted that the trial court violated his due process right to adequate competency procedures by failing to order a psychiatric evaluation with respect to his competence to stand trial.

The Supreme Court concluded that the trial court's failure to order a competency hearing violated Drope's due process right to a fair trial. Given that competency evaluations serve as procedural safeguards of the defendant's fundamental right not to be tried while incompetent, the Court determined that there is a low threshold for establishing the need for a competency hearing: "evidence of a defendant's irrational behavior, his demeanor at trial, and any prior medical opinion on competence to stand trial are all relevant in determining whether further inquiry is required, but that even one of these factors standing alone may, in some circumstances, be sufficient." The Court concluded that evidence of prior mental instability, a suicide attempt during trial, and a psychiatrist's report recommending psychiatric treatment should have been sufficient to alert the trial court to the need for further evaluation of Drope's competence to stand trial. Although the Court did not explicitly designate fixed criteria that would invariably require further inquiry, the opinion appears to encourage an inclusive interpretation of facts suggesting incompetence in order to protect the fundamental due process right not to stand trial while incompetent. The case was remanded to allow the State to retry Drope if he is found competent.

In *Godinez v. Moran*, the United States Supreme Court considered whether or not the Dusky standard applies to a defendant's competence to waive counsel and represent himself [3]. Richard Allen Moran fatally shot three people and then unsuccessfully attempted suicide. He confessed to the killings while recovering in the hospital and was charged with three counts of first-degree murder. Moran was found competent to stand trial. He subsequently moved to dismiss his attorney and to change his pleas to guilty to prevent admission of mitigating evidence at sentencing, and the trial court approved his request.

After receiving the death penalty, Moran requested relief based on the claim that he was mentally incompetent to represent himself. The 9th Circuit Court of Appeals reversed, concluding that competency to waive constitutional rights requires a heightened competency standard defined by capacity for "reasoned choice."

The Supreme Court reversed the Court of Appeals, finding that the appellate court erred in applying two different competency standards, and remanded the case. Competence to plead guilty or to voluntarily waive the right to assistance of counsel is assessed by the same *Dusky* two-prong test as competence to stand trial. The Court explicitly articulated that although states are free to adopt heightened competency requirements, the Due Process Clause only requires a standard for competence to plead guilty or waive counsel equivalent to the *Dusky* standard for competence to stand trial. The Court then clarified that, in addition to evaluating the defendant's competency, a trial court must inquire into whether the defendant's waiver of his constitutional rights was "knowing and voluntary." In this sense, according to the majority, "there *is* a 'heightened' standard for pleading guilty and for waiving the right to counsel, but it is not a heightened standard of *competence.*"

In *Indiana v. Edwards*, the United States Supreme Court faced a variation on the theme in *Godinez* – does the Constitution prohibit a state trial court from assigning counsel to a defendant who is fit to stand trial via the *Dusky* standard, if the trial court has reasons to believe the defendant may yet not be competent to represent himself?[4]

Ahmad Edwards was charged with attempted murder, battery with a deadly weapon, criminal recklessness, and theft after firing shots while attempting to steal shoes from a department store. He had a long history of schizophrenia, and his mental state became the subject of several competency hearings and self-representation requests. The present case stemmed from Edwards's request to represent himself during his retrial, which the trial court denied. Referring to his long record of psychiatric reports, the court concluded that Edwards was not competent to defend himself, even though he was competent to stand trial.

After he was convicted on the remaining counts, Edwards appealed and alleged the trial court's refusal to permit him to represent himself at his retrial deprived him of his Sixth Amendment right of self-representation.

The Supreme Court held that the Constitution permits States to require legal representation for defendants who are not mentally competent to conduct trial proceedings without the assistance of an attorney, and remanded the case for further proceedings: "[T]he Constitution permits States to insist upon representation by counsel for [defendants] competent enough to stand trial under *Dusky* but who still suffer from severe mental illness to the point where they are not competent to conduct trial proceedings by themselves."

The Supreme Court acknowledged "[m]ental illness is not a unitary concept" and interpreted this as a caution against adopting a single competency standard for different legal contexts. The Court additionally stated that a right of self-representation would not affirm the dignity of the defendant who lacks the mental capacity to proceed *pro se.* Instead, the majority found that allowing such a defendant proceed to trial without an attorney could lead to an improper conviction and, thus, "undercuts the most basic constitutional right to a fair trial." The Supreme Court, thus, held that the Constitution allows states to adopt a higher standard of competency for self-representation, and viewed trial judges as being best situated to evaluate the competency of defendants.

In a dissenting opinion, Justice Scalia, joined by Justice Thomas, provided that "the Constitution does not permit a State to substitute its own perception of fairness for the defendant's right to make his own case before the jury – a specific right long understood as essential to a fair trial." The dissent opined that if a defendant is competent to stand trial and is capable of waiving his right to counsel knowingly and voluntarily, then the defendant has a constitutional right to conduct his own defense. The dissent added that a defendant's right of self-representation should only be denied if it is necessary to allow the trial to proceed in an orderly fashion.

In *Jackson v. Indiana*, the Supreme Court considered what should be done, with regard to hospitalization and disposition of criminal charges, when a defendant is not only found incompetent to stand trial, but also not likely to be restored to fitness [5].

Theon Jackson was charged with separate robberies of two women involving a total of nine dollars. The trial court, *sua sponte*, ordered an evaluation of the defendant's mental capacity to proceed to trial given his severe cognitive, sensory, and language deficits: at age 27, Jackson was deaf, had "a mental level of a preschool child," and was unable to "read, write, or otherwise communicate except through limited sign language." At a competency hearing, two court-appointed expert psychiatrists presented uncontradicted evidence that the defendant was unable to satisfy either prong of the *Dusky* two-prong standard. They additionally opined that, due to the nature of his impairments, he was unlikely to ever develop the abilities necessary to render him competent. The trial court held that Jackson was incompetent to stand trial and ordered that he be committed to the Indiana Department of Mental Health until he is certified "sane."

Jackson moved for a new trial, contending that, given his low likelihood of ever meeting the statutory requirements for release, his pretrial commitment represented life imprisonment without ever being convicted of a crime in violation of his Fourteenth Amendment rights to due process and equal protection. The United States Supreme Court unanimously reversed, holding that Jackson's indefinite commitment exclusively due to his incompetence to stand trial violated both equal protection and due process under the Fourteenth Amendment. The Court declined to consider the issue of disposition of charges and remanded the case to the state court for further consideration and adjudication: "[A] person charged by a State with a criminal offense who is committed solely on account of his incapacity to proceed to trial cannot be held more than the reasonable period of time necessary to determine whether there is a substantial probability that he will attain that capacity in the foreseeable future. If it is determined that is not the case, then the State must either institute the customary civil proceeding that would be required to commit indefinitely any other citizen, or release the defendant."

The Supreme Court concluded that, as a matter of state law, Jackson's pretrial institutionalization was "permanent in practical effect" as the evidence sufficiently established that his chances of ever attaining the statutory competency standards were "at best minimal, if not nonexistent." It then found that the relevant Indiana statute deprived him of equal protection by subjecting him "to a more lenient commitment standard and to a more stringent standard of release than those generally applicable to all others not charged with offenses" under Indiana's civil commitment statutes. The Supreme Court additionally determined that Indiana deprived Jackson of due process by mandating continued commitment on account of his incapacity to proceed to trial despite evidence that his condition was unlikely to improve. In particular, the Court held that, "[a]t the least, due process requires that the nature and duration of commitment bear some reasonable relation to the purpose for which the individual is committed."

Performing a Capacity to Stand Trial Evaluation

Although the specific procedures for ordering and obtaining capacity to stand trial evaluations vary by jurisdiction, all potentially incompetent defendants must demonstrate that they can meet the *Dusky* standard to be deemed fit to proceed with trial. This means defendants must possess a "rational as well as factual understanding of the proceedings against him" and have the "ability to consult with [their] lawyer with a reasonable degree of rational understanding [1]."

Research and literature specific to fitness-to-stand trial in advance age populations is relatively limited. Unlike in younger populations, incompetence in an older individual may be more likely associated with symptoms of a cognitive disorder rather than active symptoms of psychosis. One study reviewed charts of 99 defendants 60 years of age or older referred for fitness-to-proceed and criminal responsibility evaluations; the authors reported that 32.1% of these defendants were found incompetent to stand trial and discussed the difficulties in treatment and restoration of competence for elderly individuals in forensic systems given the progressive and irreversible course of dementia [6].

Another study examined the specific functional impairments among patients older than 65 found unfit to stand trial compared to those found fit to stand trial [7]. Among those found not fit, the diagnosis of dementia and older age were prevalent risk factors. Deficits in orientation, memory, abstraction, concentration, calculation, and thought process were associated with incompetence, with orientation and memory correlated most strongly. With regard to specific skills implicated in lacking fitness, those with dementia had higher rates of failure to understand legal charges, potential penalties, roles of court officers, pleas, and plea-bargaining, and were unable to consult with an attorney. Most strongly correlated with incompetence to stand trial was the inability to consult with an attorney. The groups did not differ with regard to the ability to maintain appropriate courtroom behavior.

Most research has found that older age correlates inversely with time to restoration [8–14]. Not surprisingly, studies have also established that a diagnosis of dementia also predicts longer times to restoration and higher rates of unrestorability. Consistent with these findings, one study demonstrated that scores on the Repeatable Battery for the Assessment of Neuropsychological Status (RBANS) were associated with increased time to restoration [15]. Despite the above, however, a substantial number of defendants older than 65 and diagnosed with dementia are ultimately restored to fitness [13].

The trial competency evaluation for the geriatric evaluee should be approached in a manner similar to that of any other population, with attention paid to the clinical risk factors for incompetence in older age individuals as noted above. As such, the authors have utilized the American Academy of Psychiatry and the Law's Practice Guidelines for the Evaluation of Capacity to Stand Trial as the framework for discussing these assessments [16]. However, it should be noted that performing these evaluations requires specialty training and supervision. The below is intended to serve as a reference for those interested in learning more about how to assess for adjudicative competency, but it is not a substitute for the instruction required to develop expertise in this area.

Prior to the evaluation, the examiner should know why, specifically, an evaluation was requested, understand the nature of the criminal allegations against the defendant, and have an awareness of any overt history of mental illness or recent symptoms. Determination of the records necessary to review prior to the examination is dependent on the complexity of the clinical and legal issues specific to the case as they relate to the above. If there is a complicated diagnostic issue at hand, it can be useful to have recent treatment records to guide symptom review. Similarly, if there is an established history of mental illness and treatment, it can be helpful to request and review supporting documents, such has hospitalization summaries, to help characterize the presence and nature of past functional impairments stemming from psychiatric illness.

Acquiring legal paperwork such as the criminal complaint will provide the examiner with an objective understanding of the nature of the alleged offense. In addition, possessing objective documentation regarding the evidence against the defendant can aid in reality testing decision-making regarding the case. Obtaining collateral from the defense attorney regarding their relationship and exchanges with their client can be valuable in providing background on the nature of the communication, and any underlying problems, between the two parties. The patient's lawyer may also be useful in providing information regarding the evidence against the defendant. However, the examiner should refrain from solely relying or utilizing collateral obtained from the attorney, without other objective resources, for the purposes of the competency determination.

Providing the examinee with informed consent is the first essential part of the trial competency examination. This includes an explanation of the purpose of the examination and the limits of confidentiality. Similar to any informed consent process, the examiner should take steps to ensure that the individual understands the above before continuing. This maintains the ethical standard of the examination but also serves to frame the process for the defendant. The next step in the process is to perform a standard clinical review for the purposes of identifying the existence of a psychiatric illness but also to determine other nonclinical factors that may impact the way the examinee may engage with their attorney and legal system.

The clinical portion of the interview should begin with obtaining a full psychosocial history. This includes basic information on background and upbringing, traumatic experiences, relationships, education, and work history. This material will provide the examiner with insight into a subject's educational capabilities, nature of how they relate to others, and functional status. These data can be compared to evidence obtained other objective records to assess for the potential for malingering and/or an underlying cognitive disorder. The next part of the clinical interview should focus on obtaining information on past psychiatric history, substance history, medical history, and family history, following the standard guidelines for a psychiatric diagnostic assessment, and with a particular focus on neurocognitive disorders.

After obtaining the above, the examiner should complete a full review of systems and a mental status examination. Cognitive screenings include the MMSE or the MOCA, depending on clinical necessity. By the end of the clinical portion of the interview, the examiner should have an understanding of the potential differential diagnosis of underlying personality and interpersonal functioning, the possibility for any underlying psychiatric/medical issues, and an understanding of current symptoms (including those associated with cognitive functioning) as they relate to an existing or potential diagnosis. The examiner should also have a sense of whether and what they will require with regard to collateral materials/information or additional testing to clarify outstanding diagnostic questions. Given the clear relationship between neurocognitive status and fitness in older populations, the clinical interview should be performed in this age group with a focus on ruling in or out these disorders.

The second portion of the interview should focus on the legal components of the defendant's history and issues specific to trial competency. Obtaining a longitudinal criminal history can be useful in developing expectations for an individual's familiarity with the criminal justice system. It can also be helpful with establishing patterns of decision-making to compare or contrast to the current legal situation.

As noted above, determining whether an individual has the capacity to stand trial involves assessing two major functional areas: competency to assist counsel and the defendant's ability to make rational decisions regarding their case. This assessment includes having a basic understanding of legal and courtroom procedures. Because the capacity assessment is case-specific, however, the defendant must demonstrate an understanding of his/her legal predicament that is beyond general information. In addition, the examiner must also separate an individual's ignorance about aspects of the criminal justice system or their case from an inability to make a rational decision about the above. This requires that the capacity assessment process involves education around any deficits and then repeat inquires around these subjects to ensure consolidation and integration of information. For this reason, it is important that the examiner has, at the minimum, a basic understanding of the defendant's legal situation and options.

As in any capacity assessment, the focus on the interview should not only be an individual's ability to provide factual information but also to reason and appreciate the consequences of making or not making certain legal decisions and/ or providing logical reasoning for any decisions that may be against the advice of their attorney. Although providing an open-ended format for this evaluation is best, a semi-structured approach that focuses on directly assessing basic knowledge regarding criminal proceedings and the defendant's understanding of their particular case as it relates to these proceedings, followed by an assessment of their ability to work with their counsel in order to make decisions about their case and assist in their defense, is often utilized. See Appendix I for recommendations on specific areas of focus, taken from the 2007 AAPL guidelines.

Similar to evaluation of competence to make treatment decisions with regard to medical care, the determination of whether an individual has decisional capacity with regard to their legal case should connect capacity-specific functional issues to clinical observations. As such, the opinion of the evaluator, if the defendant is found unfit to stand trial, should not only highlight functional deficits with regard to thinking around their legal case but also link this to specific clinical signs and symptoms. This will additionally provide treatment targets for restoration. If a patient is found fit, the focus of the opinion should be to describe the ways in which the patient is competent, with a particular focus in addressing the issues which led to the order of the capacity evaluation.

Conclusion

A series of U.S. Supreme Court cases outlined the legal requirements regarding capacity to stand trial for defendants in criminal court. This includes *Dusky v. U.S.*, which served to define the elements of trial capacity; *Drope v. Missouri,* in which the Court recognized that trial capacity may fluctuate over time and that court has a responsibility to remain vigilant to any changes in this ability; and *Jackson v. Indiana*, which provided instruction on how to approach individuals who are unlikely to be restored to fitness. Although trial capacity evaluations in geriatric defendants should be handled in the same manner as any other individual, it is important to consider clinical phenomenon associated with advanced age, including the presence and functional implications of cognitive deficits, when performing these assessments. In addition, it is necessary that the examiner has a basic understanding of the legal process and facts related to a defendant's criminal case in order to fully assess and differentiate an evaluee's need for education from an inability to make rational decisions regarding their case.

Appendix I [16]

- Ability to provide a rational and consistent account of the alleged offense
- Knowledge about the roles of principal courtroom personnel
- Awareness of being charged with a crime and facing prosecution
- Knowledge of specific charges, the meanings of those charges, and associated penalties
- Knowledge about what specific actions the state alleges
- Ability to behave properly during court proceedings and at trial
- Capacity to appraise the impact of evidence that could be used
- Understanding of available pleas and their implications, including plea bargaining
- Perceptions and expectations of defense council
- Description of the quality and quantity of previous interactions with defense counsel
- The defendant's capacity for and willing to engage in appropriate, self-protective behavior
- The defendant's ability to retain and apply new information effectively
- The defendant's capacity to pay attention at trial and remember what has occurred
- The defendant's capacity to use information to make reasonable decisions related to his defense
- Whether the defendant has sufficient impulse control to maintain proper courtroom decorum

References

1. *Dusky v. U.S.*, 362 U.S. 402 (1960).
2. *Drope v. Missouri*, 420 U.S. 162 (1975).
3. *Godinez v. Moran*, 509 U.S. 389 (1993).

4. *Indiana v. Edwards*, 554 U.S. 164 (2008).
5. *Jackson v. Indiana*, 406 U.S. 715 (1972).
6. Lewis CF, Fields C, Rainey E. A study of geriatric forensic evaluees: who are the violent elderly? J Am Acad Psychiatry Law. 2006;34(3):324–32.
7. Frierson RL, Shea SJ, Shea ME. Competence-to-stand-trial evaluations of geriatric defendants. J Am Acad Psychiatry Law. 2002;30(2):252–6.
8. Colwell LH, Gianesini J. Demographic, criminogenic, and psychiatric factors that predict competency restoration. J Am Acad Psychiatry Law. 2011;39(3):297–306.
9. Nicholson RA, McNulty JL. Outcome of hospitalization for defendants found incompetent to stand trial. Behav Sci Law. 1992;10(3):371–83.
10. Nicholson RA, Barnard GW, Robbins L, Hankins G. Predicting treatment outcome for incompetent defendants. Bull Am Acad Psychiatry Law. 1994;22(3):367–77.
11. Rodenhauser P, Khamis HJ. Predictors of improvement in maximum security forensic hospital patients. Behav Sci Law. 1988;6(4):531–42.
12. Renner M, Newark C, Bartos BJ, McCleary R, Scurich N. Length of stay for 25,791 California patients found incompetent to stand trial. J Forensic Leg Med. 2017;51:22–6.
13. Morris DR, Parker GF. Effects of advanced age and dementia on restoration of competence to stand trial. Int J Law Psychiatry. 2009;32(3):156–60.
14. Warren JI, Chauhan P, Kois L, Dibble A, Knighton J. Factors influencing 2,260 opinions of defendants' restorability to adjudicative competency. Psychol Public Policy Law. 2013;19(4):498.
15. Toofanian Ross P, Padula CB, Nitch SR, Kinney DI. Cognition and competency restoration: using the RBANS to predict length of stay for patients deemed incompetent to stand trial. Clin Neuropsychol. 2015;29(1):150–65.
16. Mossman D, Noffsinger SG, Ash P, Frierson RL, Gerbasi J, Hackett M, Lewis CF, Pinals DA, Scott CL, Sieg KG, Wall BW. AAPL practice guideline for the forensic psychiatric evaluation of competence to stand trial. J Am Acad Psychiatry Law. 2007;35(Suppl 4):S3–72.

Chapter 14
Responding to Crisis of Aging People in Prison: Global Promising Practices and Initiatives

Tina Maschi and Adriana Kaye

Introduction

The "aging prisoner" crisis continues to gain international attention. The high human, social, and economic costs of warehousing older adults with complex physical, mental health, social, and spiritual care needs in prison continue to rapidly increase at a disproportionate rate compared to the general prison population [1, 2]. The United States has the largest number of incarcerated people aged 55 and older and that population has grown 282% between 1981 and 2011 compared to 42% in the general prison population [1]. In contrast, Canada has the lowest percentage increase in which incarcerated people aged 50 and older increased 9% in 1996 to 16% in 2005 [2]. Although there are some overlapping

T. Maschi (✉) · A. Kaye
Fordham University Graduate School of Social Services,
New York, NY, USA
e-mail: tmaschi@fordham.edu; akaye5@fordham.edu

© Springer Nature Switzerland AG 2019   219
M. Balasubramaniam et al. (eds.), *Psychiatric Ethics in Late-Life Patients*, https://doi.org/10.1007/978-3-030-15172-0_14

similarities with younger counterparts, understanding the unique developmental rights and needs of older adults will assist in the development of a geriatric-specific approach in the criminal justice system.

According to the United Nations, "older prisoners," including those with mental and physical disabilities, and terminal illnesses, are a special needs population and thus subject to special international health, social, economic practice, and policy considerations [2]. Many societies view the age of 65 as older because that is when most individuals are eligible to receive full pension or social security benefits. However, this age designation is not uniform across the world because age has different meanings in various cultures [2]. Similarly, the age at which a prisoner is defined as "older" or "elderly" varies across different countries. For example, although it varies among states, incarcerated persons in the United States may be classified as "older adult" or "elderly" as low as age 50 [1]. Other countries, such as the United Kingdom, designate age 60–65 as older. Canada has a two-tiered system in which older in prison is age 50–64 years and elderly is aged 65 and above [2].

This 50-year-old lower age classification as "elderly" in corrections is possibly because the average incarcerated person may experience accelerated decrements in their health status equivalent to community-dwelling adults who are 10–15 years older [3]. This process of accelerated aging is corroborated by international prison studies that show older adults in prison have significantly higher rates of physical and mental health decline compared to younger prisoners or older adults of a comparative age in the community [4, 5]. This rapid decline of incarcerated older adult's health has been attributed largely to their high-risk personal histories, chronic health conditions, poor health practices, such as poor diets and smoking, alcohol and substance abuse, coupled with the stressful conditions of prison confinement, such as prolonged exposure to overcrowding, social deprivation, and prison violence [6]. These combined personal and social environmental risk factors significantly increase the likelihood of the early onset of serious physical and mental illnesses, including dementia, among older adults in prison [7].

Punitive criminal justice policies have influenced this growth of the aging prison population crisis. The United States since the1980s has spearheaded the most recent "tough-on-crime" criminal justice policies, which in turn also have been adopted by many other countries [8]. For example, in the United States, stricter sentencing laws, such as "Three Strikes, You're Out," and longer mandatory prison terms have set in motion an upward trend of mass incarceration of many sentenced offenders who were destined to grow old, and even die, in overcrowded prisons [9]. More recently, countries have begun to shift to a more compassionate approach away from overly punitive policies that affect older adults in prison. For example, China passed the 2010 Criminal Law of China which bans the death penalty for people age 75 or older, except in the case of extreme homicide [10]. Currently, correctional systems across the globe, which were not designed to assume the role of long-term care facilities, are struggling with the growing wave of older adults in need of specialized care and community reintegration programming, including end-of-life care [11, 12].

In response to this crisis, over the past two decades there has been some national and international movement in corrections and the community for programs and initiatives that foster the physical, mental, social, spiritual, and economic well-being of older adults. These programs have been developed or refined in response to the recognition that older adults in prison often receive little value from prison programming that was designed for younger people in prison, such as education, vocational training, and employment programs aimed at reducing their high-risk offending behavior [13]. The need for more palliative care services is also a significant concern, given that a larger number, over 3000 (5%), of US incarcerated people, of which are mostly aged 50 or older, die every year in prison [1, 12].

To this end, this chapter reviews some of the international promising practices and programs to address the aging population in prison and post prison release. Directly following, we provide recommendations on how the professional community can assist in moving the agenda for the humanistic treatment of justice-involved older adults, including those incarcerated or formerly incarcerated.

International Promising Practices and Initiatives

Despite the challenges of managing the growing aging prison population, promising practices, initiatives, and policies have emerged across the globe that foster the health and well-being of older adults in prison. Worldwide, there are some innovative geriatric programs in prisons and post community reintegration. Promising practices often include comprehensive case management services for medical, mental health, substance abuse, family, social services, housing, education or vocational training, spiritual counseling, exercise and creative arts programs, employment, and/or retirement counseling. Program-specific aspects include one or more of the following: "age" and "cognitive capacity" sensitive environmental modifications (including the use of segregated units), interdisciplinary staff and volunteers trained in geriatric-specific correctional care, complimentary medicine, specialized case coordination, the use of family and inmate peer supports and volunteers, mentoring, and self-help advocacy group efforts.

We have classified these programs based on whether they are corrections or prison-based programs or community-based programs that provided inpatient and/or outpatient programs. Programs that serve justice-involved older adults currently across the globe. In particular, many are located in the United States (e.g., True Grit Program), the United Kingdom (e.g., RECOOP), Canada (e.g., RELIEF), and other select international locations. Please see Table 14.1 for the select programs, initiatives, and policies highlighted in this chapter.

TABLE 14.1 Programs and initiatives for justice-involved older adults: prison and community based

Corrections/prison based: inpatient or outpatient	Community based: inpatient/ outpatient
True Grit	60 West Nursing Home
The Gold Coat Program	The Aged Care and Rehabilitation Unit
The Unit for Cognitive Impairment (UCI)	Reintegration Effort for Long-term Infirm and Elderly Federal Offenders' Program (RELIEF)
NYS DOCCS Discharging Planning Unit (DPU)	Senior Ex-Offender Program (SEOP)
Chronic Disease Self-Management Education (CDSME)	Resettlement and Care for Older Ex-Offenders (RECOOP)
Long Term Offender Program (LTOP)	Project for Older Prisoners (POPS)
The Coyote Ridge Assisted-Living Unit	Families Against Mandatory Minimums (FAMM)
The Kevin Waller Unit	

Prison Corrections-Based Programs and Initiatives

Inpatient and/or Outpatient Based

Evidence suggests that older adults in prison have complex and comorbid health and mental health care needs. As a natural part of the aging process, older adults in global prison have higher rates of chronic illnesses or disabilities, such as heart and lung disease and dementia, as compared to incarcerated younger adults. Minor to serious mental health and substance abuse issues are commonplace in global prison populations, especially among older adults [14]. Perhaps, the most significant mental health issue of aging in prison is accelerated cognitive decline. Poor health behaviors coupled with the prison environment place older adults at increased risk for age-related mental health problems, especially dementia, which commonly results in the loss of physical and cognitive capacities and death [7, 15, 16]. In order to address incarcerated older adults' needs, inpatient or skilled nursing unit or geriatric-specific units, hospice programs or units, and outpatient chronic health, mental health, and social service programs have been developed internationally, especially in the United States.

Inpatient Skilled Nursing, Geriatric-Specific, and Hospice Units As listed in Table 14.1, several skilled nursing or geri-atric- or hospice-specific units were found in both the United States and other global locations, and they are reviewed below in that order, respectively.

The True Grit Program (USA) The True Grit Program in Nevada is a prison-based structured living program that attempts to foster older prisoners' well-being. The mission statement of the True Grit is "no more victims." It is set in a geriatric sociocultural environment and was designed to enhance physical health (using creative arts, recreational, and physical therapy activities), mental and social well-being (using group and individual therapy), human agency and empowerment (self-help modalities), spiritual well-being (using a prison chaplain and volunteers), and successful community reintegration (using discharge planning).

Eligibility criteria include the following:

- Being age 55 or over (with no upper age limit)
- No full-time work or school (part-time school is acceptable)
- Willingness to participate in all program activities, including correctional programs that target individual criminogenic factors
- Compliance with a signed formal contract that specifies the rules and regulations governing behavior and grooming standards

As the program developed, it became noticeable that rather than just providing a safe and healthy environment within the prison for older adults, the True Grit became a mechanism for bridging the chasm between prison and the community. It was gradually transformed into a rehabilitation and community reintegration initiative [7].

Research evidence suggests that the program is effective in increasing psychological and social well-being [17]. For instance, preliminary quantitative analysis shows 0% recidivism rates of participants who were released from prison. Qualitative data from True Grit participants suggest the program is invaluable part of their lives, helping them cope with daily prison stress while allowing them to offer restitution for their crimes [7].

- For more information about this program, go to: http://www.programsforelderly.com/cool-truegrit-prisons.php

The Gold Coat Program (California Men's Colony)- Dementia Unit Perhaps the most well-known U.S. prison dementia program is the California Men's Colony in San Luis Obispo, California. It has a dementia unit that can be described as having other inmates or "peer supports" who provide services to dying incarcerated people. This is particularly important since prisons are often dangerous environments, incarcerated with cognitive disorders become vulnerable to victimization; therefore, the availability of a hospice with peer support can be a source of protection to them [7]. The program aides consist of prisoner volunteers or "social aides" who have records of 10 years of exemplary behavior and receive training in dementia caregiving. Their responsibilities include making sure inmate patients receive medical care, provide social support, help with daily tasks, and protect them. Another interesting aspect of this program is that prisoner volunteers will receive supervision from a clinical psychologist. During supervision meetings, the clinical team address challenges such as how volunteers should respond to patients who are experiencing hallucinations. In addition, she is always available for emotional support for issues that might affect volunteers' roles such as death in the family, going through parole, or other problems [7, 18].

- For more information about this program, go to: https://www.cdcr.ca.gov/Facilities_Locator/CMC.html

The Unit for Cognitive Impairment- UCI- (Beacon, NY)-Dementia Unit Another well-known prison dementia unit is the Unit for Cognitive Impairment (UCI). The UCI is a 30-bed unit located on the third floor of the Regional Medical Unit in Fishkill Correctional Facility in New York. Currently, this is the only formal UCI in New York State; therefore, it is common for them to receive transfers from other prisons. The UCI houses individuals with health conditions that contribute to cognitive decline such as Alzheimer's disease, HIV, AIDS, TBI, Huntington's disease, and mental illnesses such as schizophrenia. The atmosphere of the unit is similar to a hospital, with all rooms having an open-door policy 24/7 unless the patient is under special supervision. Staff consists of doctors, psychiatrists, social workers, psychologists, registered nurses, nursing assistants, correction staff, and a recreational officer. Interestingly, the recreational officer acts as a liaison with community agents through the parole process. The staff strive to ensure a seamless transition for patients back to their families. The UCI administration emphasizes the importance of training for security, civilian, and clinical staff. For instance, there was an initial 40-hour training delivered by the local chapter of the Alzheimer's Association to all staff at all levels. There are also nursing educators who provide the same training to new staff and refresher courses. As part of their therapeutic care, the UCI provides patients with activities such as music, poetry, and pet therapy [7, 18].

- For more information about this program:
  - New York Tackles Inmates with Special Needs Facility: http://www.doccs.ny.gov/NewsRoom/external_news/2008-07-29_Prison_Gray.pdf

NYS DOCCS Discharging Planning Unit-DPU Currently in the New York State Department of Corrections and Community Supervision (NYS DOCCS), there is a newly established Discharge Planning Unit (DPU). The DPU consists of four nurses and one social worker who are supervised by a chief medical officer. The DPU is responsible for the discharge planning of the general population with two chronic health conditions or one serious condition. The DPU teams also work in tandem with the DOCCS medical parole coordinator to set up a discharge plan. Other individuals and organizations involved in transitional care planning include DPU staff, family members or assigned surrogates or guardian, community service providers, such as visiting nurses for home placement, or a staff member at an assisted-living or skilled nursing facility. If an individual is on parole, a parole officer also should be involved. Service providers, especially skilled nursing homes, who collaborate directly with NYS DOCCS help provide smooth care transitions, including holding a bed and having access to medical equipment needed for patients, such as wheelchairs and oxygen [19].

Outpatient Programs

In addition to prison-based inpatient type units, there are also several outpatient programs that target incarcerated older adults and/or the seriously ill. These programs include chronic disease management, community reintegration or reentry preparedness programs, and assisted-living programs. They are reviewed in the order, respectively.

Chronic Disease Self-Management Education- CDSME (Virginia) The Chronic Disease Self-Management Education (CDSME) is an evidence-based disease self-management program developed and researched by Stanford University and is administered in prison. It consists of a 6-week workshop with 2.5-hour sessions. The program offers tools and builds on skills to better deal with symptoms, manage common problems, and participate more fully in life. Long-term research shows that the program improved energy, physical activity, psychological well-being, partnerships with physicians, health status, and self-efficacy. Research findings also point out reduced fatigue, limitations on social role activities, pain symptoms, emergency room visits, hospital admissions, and hospital length of stay. In addition, national study findings also showed lower health costs and lower health care use [20, 21].

- For more information about this program, go to:
  - CDSME   Program   https://www.youtube.com/watch?v=cMYJgsB8VVM

Long Term Offender Program – LTOP (California, USA) The Long Term Offender Program (LTOP) is a voluntary program that provides services in individual and group settings. Those services address criminogenic areas such as substance use disorder, criminal thinking, anger management, family relationships, denial management, and victim impact. Individuals receiving services are offenders who are subject to the Board of Parole Hearings (BPH) parole suitability process. The program's goal is to reduce reoffending by providing cognitive behavioral treatment programming to address criminogenic needs and risks. The program is tailored according to each individual's needs, and its duration will vary accordingly. Eligibility criteria include: (a) offenders must have an assessed criminogenic need, and (b) be within 1–5 years from the BPH suitability hearing [22].

- For more information about this program, go to:
  - CDCR www.cdcr.ca.gov/rehabilitation/LTOP.html

The Coyote Ridge Assisted-Living Unit (Washington, US) The Coyote Ridge Assisted-Living Unit located in a Washington correctional facility is an assisted-living unit for incarcerated older adults and persons with disabilities. The unit has capacity to house 74 inmates who are segregated from the mainstream general prison population. They are provided with two nurses who are assigned 24 hours a day, 7 days a week. Eligibility criteria include: (a) inmates' disability and (b) minimum-security risk [23].

- For more information about this program, go to:
  - State Initiatives to Address Aging Prisoners https://www.cga.ct.gov/2013/rpt/2013-R-0166.htm

The Kevin Waller Unit (Australia) Another prison-based assisted-living unit is the Kevin Waller Unit (KWU) in Australia. KWU is for who do not require skilled nursing home type care. Operated by Correctional Services New South Wales, Australia (CSNSW) correctional, patients who do not require inpatient-based supportive care at the Aged Care and Rehabilitation Unit (see below) are transferred to the KWU. The Kevin Waller Unit has 15 beds and provides elderly offenders with independent living in segregation from the mainstream prison population [24].

For more information about this program, go to: Australia's Justice Health Website: http://www.justicehealth.nsw.gov.au/about-us/custodial-health/long-bay-hospital

Community-Based Programs and Initiatives

Inpatient Based (Skilled Nursing Homes)

In addition to prison-based programs and initiatives, there also are a number of international community-based programs that assisted incarcerated adults with community reintegration or reentry (see Table 14.1).

Inpatient (Skilled Nursing)

60 West nursing home (Connecticut, USA) The 60 West nursing home in Connecticut serves elderly, and ill residents are on nursing-home-release parole (i.e., a form of parole the state legislature created in 2013). This privately owned nursing home's mission is to specialized care, dignity, and acceptance to their residents. In order to be admitted in the nursing home, patients go through a comprehensive screening and are not accepted if they are seen to pose a risk to the public [18, 25]. This social innovation has been considered a role model for other states as it proves that a partnership between the state and privately owned organizations can be efficient at meeting the state's prison needs and be a catalyst for reforming the criminal justice system nationwide. This program has gained notoriety as the first facility in the country to gain approval from the Centers for Medicare and Medicaid Services (CMS) for federal nursing home funding, so that the needs of older incarcerated adults can be met.

- For more information about this program, go to:
  - 60 West Website: https://www.securecare-options.com/

The Aged Care and Rehabilitation Unit (Australia) The Aged Care and Rehabilitation Unit is an inpatient facility for older offenders who require long-term supported care. Operated by the Justice Health & Forensic Mental Health Network (JH & FMHN), the community-based unit is located at Long Bay Hospital, New South Wales, Australia. The Unit is equipped with 15 beds and provides palliative care to both male and female offenders. Patients receive a comprehensive assessment and treatment planning. In addition, they are also provided with daily rehabilitation-based activities such as gardening, bingo, table tennis, air hockey, and wii computer games [24].

- For more information about this program, go to:
  - Australia's Justice Health Website: http://www.justice-health.nsw.gov.au/about-us/custodial-health/long-bay-hospital

Hospices

RELIEF (Canada) The Reintegration Effort for Long-term Infirm and Elderly Federal Offenders' (RELIEF) Program was developed to facilitate the transition of elderly and infirm prisoners into the community. Established in 1999, the RELIEF program addresses the hospice care needs of elderly and infirm former prisoners (who are screened and provided hospice care training). The program was designed based on human rights and social justice values of dignity and worth of the person and respect to the dying. It also uses former prisoners and caregivers to provide compassionate peer support to fellow former inmates who are dying [26]. In other words, it provides a less institutional-like setting as clients and caregivers of the RELIEF Program are housed in four self-contained, six-bedroom houses. The facility is on ground level and accessible to wheelchairs and walkers. Clients' needs are assessed on a regular basis so that the level of intervention and support is accurately determined. Based on the assessment, they are assigned to one of three houses that offer "high," "medium," or "low" levels of attendant care [27].

- For more information about this program, access this publication:
  - http://www.csc-scc.gc.ca/publications/forum/e123/123i_e.pdf

Reentry-Focused Organizations, Programs, and Initiatives

There are several global community-based organizations and programs that address the well-being of older adults prior to and after prison released. As shown in Table 14.1, these select programs and initiatives followed by advocacy programs.

Senior Ex-Offender Program- SEOP (San Francisco, CA) The Senior Ex-Offender Program (SEOP) was the first community reintegration program in the United States to focus on the unique needs of older adults released from jails and prisons. The mission of the SEOP program is to restore self-respect. They do so by using strategies using social modeling, compassionate care, guidance, mental health, and other services. It follows the wrap-around model for connecting senior ex-offenders to services such as counseling, certified addiction specialists, behavioral health services, and basic necessities resources such as clothing and hygiene products. The program also helps senior ex-offender with transitional housing, which gives them a chance to live in the community with support systems. To qualify, individuals must be over 50 years, have been incarcerated, or are about to be released from prison. The program also assists participants with problems solving, such as helping program participants finding solutions to the challenges faced by older formerly incarcerated people. The program's goal is to give elderly formerly incarcerated people an opportunity for a new start through referrals to needed services and other social supports [28].

- For more information about this program, go to:
  - Bay View Senior Services: https://bhpms89s.org/senior-ex-offender-program/

Recoop (England) Based in England, the Resettlement and Care for Older Ex-Offenders (Recoop) is another community-based program that promotes older adults' health and well-being. It does so by providing comprehensive care, resettlement, and rehabilitation services of incarcerated and formerly incarcerated older adults. For example, the program provides support services, advocacy, financial advice, and mentoring on issues, such as employment and training. They also provide advice on housing and health that will enable them to take control of their lives and remain free from reoffending and minimizing social isolation [29].

More specifically, the RECOOP program addresses nine different pathways to rehabilitate and ultimately reduce reoffending among older adults, those are: attitudes, thinking, and behavior; accommodation; drugs and alcohol; children and families; health; education, training, and employment; finance, benefit, and debt; abuse; and prostitution. Among the different services provided, the RECOOP offers the Transition 50+ Resettlement program, which was designed to address specific resettlement needs of individuals over the age of 50. The goals are to provide justice-involved older adults with appropriate knowledge and skills to support a positive resettlement experience and prevent reoffending [30]. When it comes to program effectiveness, in 2013, the Justice Select Committee and the Prisons Inspectorate recognized the South West prison services (HMP Leyhill and HMP Dartmoor) as having good practice models [31].

- For more information about this program, go to:
  - RECOOP: http://recoop.org.uk/pages/home/

Community Advocacy and Supports

Additionally, there are community advocacy and supports in the form of programs and state and national initiatives relevance to fostering the well-being of justice-involved older adults. For example, the Project for Older Prisoners and Families Against the Mandatory Minimum.

Project for Older Prisoner- POPS (USA) The Project for Older Prisoners (POPS) is considered a policy and cultural level response to the aging prisoner crisis. It is a law school-based advocacy program to address the rights and needs of incarcerated older adults. The program is a risk-based approach to addressing the aging prisoner problem. It involves law student volunteers who assist individual low-risk prisoners older than 55 years to help them obtain paroles, pardons, or alternative forms of incarceration. When an assessment for risk of recidivism is low, students help to locate housing and support for prisoners. They also help prepare the case for a parole hearing established in 1989 at Tulane Law School and has expanded across the United States. In 2003, the POPS program suggested the expansion of its programs across the United States to the growing aging prisoner population as advocacy issues [7].

- For more information about this program, go to:
  - POPS-Project for Older Prisoners: https://elderlyrelease.wordpress.com/pops-project-fror-older-prisoners/

Families Against Mandatory Minimums-FAMM- *(Washington, D.C)* Founded in 1991, FAMM is a national advocacy organization that promotes fair and effective criminal justice reforms to make our communities safe, including compassionate release of loved ones. The organization's mission is "to create a more fair and effective justice system that respects our American values of individual accountability and dignity while keeping our communities safe." It strives to promote change through the voices of those who face unjust sentencing and its negative effects. Public education and targeted advocacy are key elements to FAMM's success to date. Since 1991, over 312,000 people have benefited from sentencing reforms championed by FAMM [32].

- For more information about this organization, go to:
  - FAMM's website: https://famm.org/about-us/

Conclusion and Next Steps

As illustrated throughout this chapter, there is growing international awareness and response to the growing population of older adults in prison. Correctional and community-based settings both locally and globally are in a unique position to address the rights and needs of the vulnerable group of elders. This chapter provides examples of promising programs and initiatives that are being implemented in corrections and community-based settings that attempt to do just that. Some useful next steps to build upon existing innovations for the professional community to consider include the following:

1. Conducting an institutional and community-based needs assessment for organizational readiness for the provision of forensic geriatric mental health and other needed services.
2. Developing or refining programs, including prison-based discharge planning units, residential facilities, especially for the older prison population with mental health issues.
3. Developing or refining staff trainings for professional that include forensic geriatric mental health assessment and treatment, including reentry preparedness.

4. Assessing and revising where warranted national and state laws that impact aging prison population, especially geriatric and compassionate release policies.

One or more of these suggested action steps can assist with continuing to build upon the momentum for providing mental health and other services for the vulnerable population of older adults involved in the criminal justice system.

References

1. Human Rights Watch. Old behind bars [Internet]. 2012. Available from: https://www.hrw.org/report/2012/01/27/old-behind-bars/aging-prison-population-united-states.
2. United Nations Office on Drugs and Crime. Handbook for prisoners with special needs. Vienna: United Nations; 2009.
3. American Civil Liberties Union. At America's expense: the mass incarceration of the elderly [Internet]. Washington, DC; 2012. Available from: http://www.aclu.org/report/americas-expense-mass-incarceration-elderly.
4. Dai W, Yu F. The correction of old prisoners: a sociological study. China Prison J. 2011;4:25–9.
5. Davies M. The integration of elderly prisoners: an exploration of services provided in England and Wales. Int J Criminol. 2011;1:1–32.
6. Stojkovic S. Elderly prisoners: a growing and forgotten group within correctional systems vulnerable to elder abuse. J Elder Abuse Negl. 2007;19(3–4):97–117.
7. Maschi T, Kwak J, Ko E, Morrissey M. Forget me not: dementia in prison. The Gerontologist. 2012;52(4):441–51.
8. Maschi T, Viola D, Sun F. The high cost of the international aging prisoner crisis: well-being as the common denominator for action. The Gerontologist. 2012;53(4):543–54.
9. Kinsella C. Correctional health care costs. Lexington: Council of State Governments; 2004.
10. Guo X. A discussion on the reform of correction system of older offenders. Hebei Law Sci. 2011;29(7):126–32.
11. Aday R. Aging prisoners. Westport: Praeger; 2003.
12. Stone K, Papadopoulos I, Kelly D. Establishing hospice care for prison populations: an integrative review assessing the UK and USA perspective. Palliat Med. 2011;26(8):969–78.

13. Mesurier R. Supporting older people in prison: ideas for practice [Internet]. Age UK; 2011. Available from: https://www.ageuk.org. uk/documents/en-gb/for-professionals/government-andsociety/ older%20prisoners%20guide_pro.pdf?dtrk=true.
14. James D, Glaze L. Mental health problems of prison and jail inmates. Rockville: U.S. Department of Justice; 2006.
15. Schoenly L. Perfect storm looming: inmate dementia is on the horizon [Internet]. CorrectionsOne. 2010 [cited 19 July 2018]. Available from: https://www.correctionsone.com/correctional-healthcare/articles/2083910-Perfect-storm-looming-Inmate-dementia-is-on-the-horizon/
16. Wilson J, Barboza S. The looming challenge of dementia in prisons. Correctional Care [Internet]. 2010 [cited 18 July 2018];24(2):10–3. Available from: http://www.ncchc.org/pubs/CC/ archive/24-2.pdf.
17. Harrison M. True grit: an innovative program for elderly inmates. Correct Today. 2006;1:46–9.
18. Brown J. Living with dementia in prison. Churchill Trust; 2015.
19. NYS Department of Corrections and Community Supervision [Internet]. Doccs.ny.gov. 2018 [cited 19 July 2018]. Available from: www.doccs.ny.gov/doccs.html.
20. National Association of Area Agencies on Aging. Supporting America's aging prisoner population: opportunities & challenges for area agencies on aging [Internet]. National Association of Area Agencies on Aging; 2017. Available from: https://www.n4a. org/Files/n4a_AgingPrisoners_23Feb2017REV%20(2).pdf.
21. Thornton E, Welch J, Holmes A. Chronic disease self-management education in Virginia's prison. Presentation presented at; Virginia; 2015.
22. Jr. E, Diaz R, Force W. Long-Term Offender Program – Division of Rehabilitative Programs [Internet]. Cdcr.ca.gov. 2018 [cited 6 July 2018]. Available from: https://cdcr.ca.gov/rehabilitation/ LTOP.html.
23. McCarthy K. State initiatives to address aging prisoners [Internet]. OLR Research Report; 2013. Available from: https:// www.cga.ct.gov/2013/rpt/2013-R-0166.htm.
24. Baldwin J, Leete J. Behind bars: the challenge of an ageing prison population. Aust J Dement Care. 2012;1(2):16–9.
25. Wisnieski A. 'Model' nursing home for paroled inmates to get federal funds [Internet]. Connecticut Health Investigative Team. 2018 [cited 19 July 2018]. Available from: http://c-hit.org/2017/04/25/ model-nursing-home-for-paroled-inmates-to-get-federal-funds/

26. APCCA Newsletter. A program that works with and treats elderly and infirm offenders in the Pacific Region, Canada [Internet]. 2000 [cited 18 October 2018]. Available from: http://www.apcca.org/Pubs/news11/#item15.

27. Stewart J. The Reintegration Effort for Long-Term Infirm and Elderly Federal Offenders (RELIEF) Program. Forum on Corrections Research. 2000;12(3).

28. Senior Ex-Offender Program [Internet]. Bayview Senior Services. 2018 [cited 18 October 2018]. Available from: https://bhpmss.org/senior-ex-offender-program/

29. Doing time: the experiences and needs of older people in prison [Internet]. Prisonreformtrust.org.uk. 2008 [cited 19 July 2018]. Available from: http://www.prisonreformtrust.org.uk/Portals/0/Documents/Doing%20Time%20the%20experiences%20and%20needs%20of%20older%20people%20in%20prison.pdf.

30. RECOOP- Resettlement and Care of Older ex-Offenders and Prisoners – Transition 50+ Resettlement [Internet]. Recoop.org.uk. 2018 [cited 19 July 2018]. Available from: http://www.recoop.org.uk/pages/services/transition-50-resettlement.php.

31. HM Chief Inspector of Prisons for England and Wales. Prisons Inspectorate. London, England: Williams Lea Group; 2013.

32. About Us | FAMM [Internet]. FAMM. 2018 [cited 18 October 2018]. Available from: https://famm.org/about-us/.

Index